"Lele's *The Baby and the Biome* is a wonderful response to the surprising and life-threatening atopic episodes that Lele, and increasingly many others, encounter with their children. This is the book for parents wondering why eczema, food allergies, and asthma have become a modern epidemic, and what we can do to stop them."

—Michael Brandwein, PhD, lecturer at the Hebrew University of Jerusalem and CTO and cofounder of MYOR Diagnostics

THE BABY
and
THE BIOME

....

How the Tiny World
Inside Your Child Holds
the Secret to Their Health

....

Meenal Lele

with Sarah Durand

Foreword by Cezmi Akdis, MD

AVERY

An imprint of Penguin Random House

New York

AVERY

an imprint of Penguin Random House LLC
penguinrandomhouse.com

Most Avery books are available at special quantity discounts for bulk purchase for
sales promotions, premiums, fund-raising, and educational needs. Special books
or book excerpts also can be created to fit specific needs. For details, write:
SpecialMarkets@penguinrandomhouse.com.

Library of Congress Cataloging-in-Publication Data
has been applied for.

9780593421024 (hardcover)
9780593421031 (ebook)

Printed in the United States of America
1st Printing

BOOK DESIGN BY KATY RIEGEL

Neither the publisher nor the author is engaged in rendering professional
advice or services to the individual reader. The ideas, procedures, and
suggestions contained in this book are not intended as a substitute for
consulting with your physician. All matters regarding your health
require medical supervision. Neither the author nor the publisher
shall be liable or responsible for any loss or damage allegedly
arising from any information or suggestion in this book.

To my boys. Who are the reason for everything.

Contents

Foreword

Allergies, autoimmune diseases, and neurodegenerative diseases have been rising at an alarming rate since the 1960s. This rise has coincided with the introduction of new chemicals that have caused catastrophic damage to the earth and human health. A growing body of data suggests that damage to the human epithelial barrier (skin, gut, and lungs), together with changes in the microbiomes of these areas, is contributing to food allergy, eczema, asthma, environmental allergies, celiac disease, inflammatory bowel disease, and other conditions. Leakiness of the gut epithelium (or "leaky gut") and decreased biodiversity in the gut microbiome are connected to autoimmune and metabolic conditions such as diabetes, obesity, multiple sclerosis, rheumatoid arthritis, lupus, ankylosing spondylitis, and autoimmune hepatitis. Finally, inflammatory responses due to a "leaky gut" and microbiome changes are even suspected in Alzheimer's disease, Parkinson's disease, chronic depression, stress-related psychiatric disorders, and autism spectrum disorders.

The "epithelial barrier hypothesis" has emerged as an over-arching explanation for the increase in disease. This relatively new hypothesis proposes that skin / gut / lung tissue defects, triggered by exposure to toxic substances, are the starting point of many immune diseases. While genetics play a part, environmental exposures have a bigger role. A leaky epithelial barrier allows microbes to move from the surface of affected tissues to inside the tissue and even deeper. This movement by opportunistic pathogens causes a cascade of inflammation, reshapes the microbiome, and leaves it in a perpetually pro-inflammatory state.

We have long known that many environmental substances can damage the epithelial barriers and cause microbial dysbiosis, or an imbalance of the microbiome. These include laundry and dish-washer detergents, cosmetics, household cleaning products, enzymes, preservatives, and emulsifiers in processed food, cigarette smoke, particulate matter, diesel exhaust, ozone, nanoparticles, and microplastics. Recent studies indicate that the barrier-damaging effect of these substances, even at low concentrations, can be further aggravated by existing chronic inflammation.

In this book, Meenal Lele, the mother of two children, shares her journey of caring for her son Leo, who suffers from severe allergies. She sees the big picture and carries her maternal experience and extensive research to everyone involved, including the patients themselves, their parents, doctors, nurses, and dieticians. Throughout the course of this book, *The Baby and the Biome*, the author explores the development of her son Leo's conditions, manifested as immune diseases, food allergy, environmental allergies, and eczema. She connects the dots between her son's complex symptoms, microbiome alterations, and environmental exposures. This proved a challenging task, as most doctors and patients focus on treating the disease itself, taking little consideration of its triggers and preventive measures.

Meenal Lele's research and experience are shared in this book in a very warm writing style, and it is an invaluable reference, not only for parents caring for children with the chronic conditions listed above but also for adults with these conditions.

I also highly recommend *The Baby and the Biome* for doctors to share with patient families and medical students at the beginning of their studies. Real-life examples and anecdotes make this book a must-read for all parents preparing to have a child. It is an essential guide for parents on early baby care, antibiotics, diet recommendations, the impact of the environment on health, and nurturing the pre- and postnatal biome of the baby. *The Baby and the Biome* covers practical preventative measures such as good bathing tips, birthing practices, skin protection, reducing exposure to environmental toxins in air pollution, detergents, and protection of the gut microbiome through diet. In a concerted effort by Leo's parents to restore the function of his epithelial barriers, he has gone from taking several daily medications to none.

Allergies, autoimmune diseases, and neurodegenerative diseases affect almost two billion patients worldwide, and their prevalence continues to rise. The continuously growing epidemic has developed at the same time as the introduction, with limited governmental regulations, of almost 200,000 new chemicals to human lives. While written for parents, this book should be considered a major reference for regulatory authorities and politicians to better understand the daily life of patients and their families and guide their new policies toward a greener and healthier world.

Cezmi Akdis, MD
March 2022

Overview of My Son's Immune Disease Development

Throughout the course of this book, I will trace the development of my son Leo's immune diseases and describe how they manifested themselves. Many parents struggle to connect the dots between their child's multiple and various symptoms, and I was no different. When children break out into rashes, have an asthma attack, or worse, end up in the emergency room because they are vomiting profusely after ingesting peanuts, parents may become so focused on the urgent situation at hand that they don't think about all the other conditions and factors that played into it.

The diagram on the next page lays out how Leo's conditions began, then continued, then cascaded into what felt like an out-of-control series of problems that kept getting worse. When I talk about what Leo went through—and often still endures to this day—I'm often reminded of something called *structured criticality*. This principle states that small, seemingly insignificant factors can trigger momentous, often catastrophic change because of the interrelatedness of all the elements that make up the situation. Think of a mountain of sand. As you pour more sand on top, you create an organized, symmetric cone. But as the mountain gets bigger and bigger, it becomes unstable, and then something as tiny as a single grain of sand added to the pile can set off an avalanche that destroys everything in its path.

This book will help you prevent that avalanche. Through my story and my research, I will untangle the nature and relatedness of immune diseases so you can learn how to tackle the root cause of your child's symptoms. I hope that by seeing how Leo's conditions originated and are connected, you can create a better life for your child, your family, and your future children.

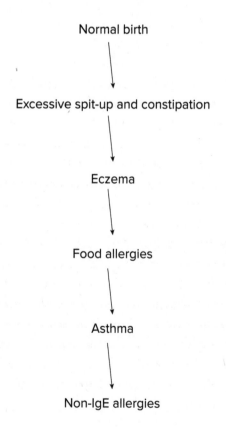

Normal birth

Excessive spit-up and constipation

Eczema

Food allergies

Asthma

Non-IgE allergies

Introduction

In September 2016, I spent the day before my thirty-third birthday concerned and confused about my two-and-a-half-year-old son's "cold."

Leo had woken up that Sunday morning with a runny nose, the rattly sound of chest congestion, and a general sense of lethargy. My husband, Scott, and I fed breakfast to him and our ten-month-old son, Kaden, then got both boys dressed and began to plan the morning.

Instead of being excited at the idea of going to the playground as he usually was, Leo stayed on the couch, halfheartedly playing with his toys. *Wow, this cold is bad,* I thought. Scott and I looked at each other, sad our little guy was feeling so crummy, and decided to leave him be. While Scott put on a jacket, I strapped Kaden into his stroller. Then I kissed them both goodbye and locked the door behind them as they headed outside into the beautiful fall sunshine. I walked back to the couch and sat down with Leo.

He didn't seem to be up for much besides watching cartoons. For the next hour, Leo started to seem better. His breathing was still short, but his temperature didn't rise above normal and his occasional coughs never turned into spasms. Every now and then, though, I noticed his chest retract in a strange way, like it was sinking just a little too deeply and a little too hard. It seemed weird to me, and I took a video on my iPhone, but it didn't happen consistently, so I wasn't overly concerned. I stroked his curls and tried to reassure him that I was there.

One cartoon turned into three, and Scott returned with Kaden so he could put him down for a nap.

"How's Leo doing?" he asked as he hung up his jacket and unstrapped Kaden.

"He's okay," I said, trying to sound confident. "He's still really low energy, but he seems a little better when I lie down on the couch with him. It's definitely a nasty chest cold. He probably caught it at day care."

I fed Leo an early lunch and worried just a little bit when he didn't finish it. Leo was always hungry, so this wasn't like him. Then I scooped him up and carried him to his room so he could take his afternoon nap. After he went down, I briefly considered calling his pediatrician. Part of me was sure they would tell me I was overreacting, but another part of me had a nagging feeling this was more than a cold. Almost immediately I decided against doing this because it was the weekend.

As I walked to the kitchen to make my own lunch, I noticed Scott sitting down at his computer. I pulled up a chair next to him. "Can you google 'toddler strained breathing' or something like that?" I asked. "Maybe 'toddler cold with cough'? I just want to make sure this is only a cold."

"Sure," he answered, then started to type. Page after page of content popped up on the screen, and we skimmed it together for the next ten minutes or so. Everything we saw was vague and unhelpful, and Scott closed his computer. "Let's call my brother after dinner," he suggested. "He's a pulmonologist. He'll know what to do."

After Leo woke up and returned to the couch to watch cartoons, Scott and I spent the afternoon watching over him like any concerned parent would. At dinner, we traded worried glances as Leo picked at his food and Kaden devoured his. After we cleaned up the dishes and took the boys to the living room so they could play, we FaceTimed Scott's brother. When he picked up, we chatted a little bit, then dove into details of how Leo had been feeling all day. We carried the phone into the living room so my brother-in-law could see Leo and say hi.

He took one look at our son and cleared his throat. "I think he's having an asthma attack," he said. "You should take him to the nearest ER right away."

Scott scooped Kaden up, and I got Leo. We rushed toward the door, slipped on our boys' shoes, and put their jackets on as gently as we could. Then we carried Kaden and Leo to the car, jumped in, and sped the five miles to the Children's Hospital of Philadelphia. Scott dropped Leo and me at the entrance while he and Kaden went to park.

Leo did *not* want to go through those hospital doors. He had visited the hospital a year before for a reaction to an undiagnosed egg allergy, and he clearly remembered it. He screamed bloody murder, and I carried him through the sliding doors and into the line, unsure of what I was going to say to whomever was going to check me in. After all, nothing was *really* wrong with him, right?

When I reached the triage desk, a nurse looked up slowly, ready to deal with yet another crying child and overdramatic parent. Then she saw my son and sprang up from her chair.

"Child in respiratory distress!" she yelled as she looked over her shoulder toward another nurse. "Let's get a bed *now*."

"He's been like this all day . . ." I answered, as if it were my job to calm *her* down, not the other way.

Instead, she began prodding me. "Why didn't you bring him in sooner?!" she demanded. "His lungs could have shut down, and he could have died."

I stepped back, stung by her incriminatory tone. Then a tech approached me and took Leo from my arms, and I watched in a daze as a team of doctors and nurses rushed him to a room, laid him on a bed, and put an oxygen mask on him.

Leo was screaming the whole time.

"Ninety percent oxygen levels," one of the nurses said to no one in particular. Then she turned to me. "We're going to give your son inhaled steroids to bring his oxygen levels back to normal."

One of the doctors turned to me. "I can't believe his oxygen is that low," he commented. "He shouldn't be able to cry that much!"

I don't recall if a few minutes or an hour passed, but things settled down, and the clatter of instruments and buzz of machines faded into background noise. At some point a nurse pulled me aside to ask me about Leo's medical history and medications.

"Well," I answered as she began to type notes into a computer, "he was diagnosed with eczema when he was six months old. He's also allergic to peanuts, eggs, and all tree nuts. But this is just a bad cold he caught at day care." I smiled and shrugged. "You know how these viruses go around!"

The nurse gave me an incredulous look. "Didn't you know he could develop severe asthma because of his food allergies?" she asked.

I guess, I thought. *Sort of.*

At that time I worked as the head of clinical research for a medical device company, and I spent my days immersed in the latest advancements in science. I had read dozens of studies on childhood allergies since Leo's eczema diagnosis had led us to test him for food allergies as a possible cause, but somehow any mention of asthma had slipped right past me. (We often ignore information we don't want to know.) My biggest issue, though, was that I didn't know what an asthma attack looked like. No one I knew had asthma. I didn't have the faintest idea that the weird breathing Leo had been doing on and off all day was a classic sign of a childhood asthma attack, or that his breathing "too deeply" was called *neck tugging*. I was also confused enough about asthma to think an attack could be triggered only by fumes, smoke, or exercise—not by a common cold.

The nurse shook her head as I snapped back into reality. "I'm sorry, but asthma is serious," she said, "and it could have killed your son."

Leo didn't die that night, of course. The inhaled steroids relieved his constricted airways, and as his oxygen levels rose, his breathing became normal. Because the doctor wanted Leo to last two hours without needing another dose of medication, we stayed overnight. I hardly slept, and I'm not sure Leo did, either. Every hour a doctor would wake him for more testing. The next morning—my birthday—Scott left Kaden with my parents and came to the hospital at visiting hours. After he gave me a change of clothes and wrapped Leo in a hug, we walked to another floor to attend a class on asthma management. The instructor was kind and reassuring, telling us that while asthma could be deadly, it was also incredibly common and manageable. Children could live full, healthy lives by treating the disease with daily inhaled steroids.

Daily steroids?

Over the two and a half years of Leo's life thus far, I had come to terms with his eczema. Though his occasional red, itchy flares were hard to look at, the steroid cream we applied to them largely solved the problem, and I knew that almost 30 percent of children had eczema. I had even accepted his food allergies. They, too, were common, and we could control them by avoiding his food triggers.

But asthma that needed steroids every day to keep his lungs breathing? That really hurt. Taking life-sustaining medicine *forever* had no part in the dreams I had for my son. I suddenly felt like Leo's health and future were slipping out of control, and I worried that if he kept developing new conditions, what might he develop next?

I couldn't let him live like that.

The hospital discharged Leo that day, and when we got home, Scott took a deep breath and expressed relief that the episode was behind us. But I was even more frustrated than I'd been in the asthma management class. Scott and I had seen a geneticist when I was pregnant, and she had assured us our baby had no genetic risk of *any* disease. My family was from India, my husband's from Germany and Ireland, so we shared no recessive genes. Neither of us had a family history of any major illness, either. I'd eaten well and exercised during my pregnancy. I'd had a "normal" birth. After Leo and I got home from the hospital, we'd seen the pediatrician on schedule, and I'd taken notes and created calendar reminders for my son's vaccinations and developmental milestones. I read books, listened to podcasts, and did everything a good parent was supposed to do, including breastfeeding, washing Leo daily, waiting three days between trying new foods, and keeping him out of the sun. Our son *should* have been healthy.

But somehow I had almost killed him.

Where had I gone wrong? And where had others? If his asthma was such a strong possibility because of his allergies, why hadn't anyone shown me what to look for? Where were all the doctors and experts airing podcasts and writing articles about the fact that a potentially fatal asthma attack could be triggered by something as relatively unimportant as a cold? More than that, why hadn't anyone helped me *prevent* his asthma if we knew it was coming?

As I sat and stewed in my kitchen that day, I acknowledged that this was a question that had been nagging at me in the back of my mind for a long time.

....

The Beginning of
My Search for Answers

A year and a half earlier, it was March 2015, and Leo was eleven months old. He was a happy little boy who had just started walking, and Scott and I were thrilled that I'd recently found out I was pregnant again. We were also relieved that we had finally gotten Leo's eczema under control through steroid creams, and we were both looking forward to the "cake smash" picture we wanted to take on his first birthday. The cake recipe called for eggs, and because I am a preparer, I decided he had better try some before then. One Sunday morning I gave him a scrambled egg for breakfast. A few minutes after he devoured it, the skin around his mouth began to turn red. Within twenty minutes he had hives all over his body.

Instead of rushing Leo to the ER, Scott and I sat there confused. When he was tested for food allergies the month before, the allergist found him to be allergic to peanuts—but not eggs. How in the world had he developed an egg allergy?

After a stupid amount of hemming and hawing, Scott and I finally took Leo to the ER, where they put him on a bunch of monitors and gave him oral steroids. A few hours later, we were able to bring him home and put him to sleep in his crib.

As I mentioned before, I worked in the medical field, and to stay on top of research that might affect my work, I made a point of regularly reading *The New England Journal of Medicine*. Less than a week after Leo's allergic reaction to eggs, I opened the *Journal* up on my computer and noticed an article about the Learning Early About Peanut Allergy (LEAP) study.[1] As I stared at my screen, I couldn't believe what I was reading. The LEAP study claimed that 80 percent of (four out of five) peanut allergies in babies with eczema or an egg allergy could be *prevented* by simply feeding peanuts to babies.

This finding was *the exact opposite* of what our doctor had told us to do. When Leo was born, the prevailing recommendation was still that babies should avoid peanuts until age two because feeding them earlier would *cause* a peanut allergy. Now here was scientific proof that I could have prevented one of Leo's food allergies. I might have stopped a lifetime of worrying about accidental exposure to peanuts; I could have packed peanut butter and jelly sandwiches in his lunch box; and I could have avoided the upset I was already feeling about his having to sit at the "allergy table" in his elementary school lunchroom. (Mind you, at this point he was three years away from kindergarten, but concerns about your child's being an outcast don't follow a timeline.)

If only I had known.

I kept coming back to the LEAP study again and again over the next few weeks. I pored through the data tables and downloaded every paper referenced by the authors as well as the papers the references cited. I wrote down the key points of the

LEAP study, and what we had done wrong, to share with my husband. We had another child on the way, and I was not going to make the same mistakes twice.

As I read, my mind kept circling around the same questions. How could doctors have been so wrong? Was it true that no study had ever been done to support the "wait until age two" feeding recommendation? And when Leo developed eczema around six months old, why didn't anyone explain that eczema can cause food allergies? This connection was obviously known, since the LEAP study used "presence of severe eczema" to define "high risk of peanut allergy," and the LEAP study had started five years ago.

Life got busy after that, and I pushed my detective work off to the side. Scott and I continued to do our best to avoid Leo's allergic triggers, and we treated his eczema when it flared up. I gave birth to Kaden in November 2015, used the knowledge I'd gained from the LEAP study to help him avoid developing the allergies that plagued his brother, and settled into a life defined by the chaos of kids and a full-time job but rounded out by love.

Then in September 2016, Leo went to the hospital for the asthma attack I'd never expected he would have.

I lay in bed one night a few weeks after that attack, unable to shake the feeling that I was missing something. I decided to get up, go downstairs, and open my notebook. In engineering school, we were taught to solve problems by asking "Why?" until you got to a fundamental truth, and I applied that strategy here.

Problem: Leo had been hospitalized.

Why?

He had an asthma attack.

Why?

His lungs constrict when he gets chest colds.

Why?

His immune system is overactive.

Why?

His immune system is being stimulated when it shouldn't be. So far, all obvious. But *why?*

For some reason, I thought back on the LEAP study research I'd done a year and a half before and remembered one of many papers that had looked deeper into its findings. That paper was an attempt to find differences between the children who prevented allergies with early introduction and those who didn't, and it mentioned how *Staphylococcus aureus* skin infections in eczema could trigger a food allergy response.

I did a quick text search of all the papers I had saved on my computer and found that every single one published since 2014—and many before—talked about the role of the skin barrier and the microbiome (the tiny world of bacteria, fungi, protozoa, and viruses that exist in and on your body) in allergic diseases. Was it possible that a barrier dysfunction, coupled with a disruption of the microbiome, could be causing the tidal wave of problems my son was having? Could it be that if there wasn't a strong enough barrier in his lungs, in his gut, and on his skin, unwanted things might have found their way into his body, triggering an overactive immune system? Or could it be the opposite, that a disruption of the microbiome broke down his barriers and let food leak into places it shouldn't? According to everything I was reading, it kinda didn't matter. His barriers, his microbiome, and my son's immune conditions went hand in hand in hand.

Every paper talked about the role of the skin barrier and the microbiome in allergic diseases.

I felt like I had stumbled on a hidden secret, but I wasn't sure. So I did what I had always done in my career. I started asking questions. I spoke to dozens of doctors, pediatric nurses, research scientists, and nutritionists. I read hundreds of research papers that spanned veterinary medicine, immunology, bacteriology, genealogy, and nutrition science. When I was done, I realized that *doctors and scientists were converging on a deep systemic explanation for childhood immune diseases that no one was talking about with parents like me.*

....

I Wrote This Book to Show You That Allergies Are Not Random

In the next chapter, I'll explain allergic and immune diseases, show how they are triggered by weakened skin, gut, and lung barriers, and lay out the microbiome's key role in our barriers. For now, understand that my search for answers has shown me that the problems children like Leo face are much bigger than just food allergies. Like me, every parent I have spoken to about allergies, eczema, or asthma eventually opens up about other "weird" things about their child's temperament, pooping, and more that they secretly suspect is related. There is clearly much more to the story of allergic disease than doctors let on, and patients have not been educated or given the tools to deal with them. Immune disease needs a revolution in thinking—and an accessible way for parents to understand it.

My goal is for this book to lead that revolution.

Since late 2016, I have committed myself to trying to understand what happened to my son. Beyond the conversations with doctors and literature searches, I've joined Facebook groups, followed blogs, and posted on message boards. I've helped friends who want to understand their children's allergic diseases and work to prevent future reactions, and—standing at the playground or in the school pickup line—I've answered what feels like a million questions about the science I've learned. In 2018,

I even started a company, Lil Mixins, to educate parents about how to prevent their children from developing allergic diseases.

We are all making the same mistakes. When my older son fell sick, I didn't think twice about asking for an antibiotic, an anti-reflux medication, or a fever reducer to make him feel better. And some of the doctors who wrote the prescriptions didn't try to stop me. In this book, I'll show how destructive antibiotics can be and how they can set off a cascade of disease. Likewise, I delivered both my boys vaginally, then breastfed, but I never once thought about the quality of the microbiome that I was passing to them during their birth or through breast milk. And again, not one person or book at the time suggested that I think about it.

Baby books advised me to wash my babies daily, wait three days between trying new foods, and keep them out of the sun at all costs. These recommendations are not backed by science, and every single one (and many more) that I followed religiously can actively hurt your child by depriving them of healthy bacteria, healthy diet diversity, and essential vitamin D—all of which can reduce the risk of allergic diseases.

The list goes on. Most doctors will prescribe a steroid to control eczema before trying diet and environmental modification to treat the underlying cause and keep the immune system from attacking the skin. And five whole years after the LEAP study proved that feeding babies peanuts early and often trains the immune system to regulate, a 2020 self-reported survey showed that most pediatricians are still not telling parents to do so.[2] This one intervention could stop hundreds of thousands of kids from developing a lifelong immune condition.

With my second son, I had learned many of my mistakes and was able to fix them. Today I have two sons, born with the same genetic inputs into the same household. Yet the older one has ten food allergies, eczema, asthma, IBD, and emotional regulation issues, while my younger son is simply healthy. One son requires preplanned or premade meals and a bag of medicine everywhere we go. With the other child we can simply walk out the door and see where the day takes us.

The goal of this book is to give you a new way of caring for yourself and your baby by prioritizing the microbiome and protecting its delicate barriers. I will explore the paradigm shifts brought on by thinking about immune disease as one giant bucket of conditions, demystify the concept of the microbiome and its relationship to barrier dysfunction, and open a window so that you can see yourself and your baby for what you are: superorganisms, both human and microbe. I will then unveil a more informed approach to the ABCDEs of a baby's first thousand days: antibiotic use, baby care, diet, and environment. These components working together are the primary determinants of a healthy microbiome, barrier, and baby.

I realize that most parents are like me in that they don't seriously tackle a problem until it's right in front of them. I certainly didn't think about the biome, barriers, and immune disease when I was pregnant with Leo. I began to consider these issues only once he got sick

The goal of this book is to give you a new way of caring for yourself and your baby by prioritizing the microbiome and protecting its delicate barriers.

and I had a second child on the way. Most readers need information about what they can do for their suddenly sick toddlers *right now*, so I will begin this book a few months after birth and then dive into pregnancy and your baby's birth in later chapters. In time, though, I hope that parents will start to think about immune issues *before* they become pregnant. Perhaps this book and my story will help change that.

It is important to understand that even as I write this, new scientific information about the biome, immune disease, and barriers is being released at a rapid pace. I will explore what doctors and scientists have uncovered today and what that understanding implies about how parents can protect their children. Everything presented in this book is published in medical journals, addressed in pediatric and OB-GYN practice guidelines, and sanity-checked with leading doctors. But please understand that the research is in its baby years (pun intended!) and recommendations from doctors will undoubtedly evolve as they dig deeper. In order to avoid leading parents astray, I will focus on the things that have the biggest impact and that doctors and scientists feel are unlikely to change.

Babies are like new gardens waiting to teem with life. Whether each garden will eventually have grasses or trees, what kinds of birds will make their homes in that garden, and which worms will be in the dirt are all based on a dizzying number of variables. Trying to control which seeds the wind or animals will carry in is impossible. You'll never be able to predict with certainty if an invasive beetle will find its way in or just how much rain this piece of land will get.

But you can be sure that allowing massive fires, dumping drums of industrial waste, or letting deer eat up all the plants will all be bad for your wildflower garden. The garden will live, but it will definitely be less healthy.

In this same way, you will never be able to fully control your baby's health. It depends on way too many things. Even so, there are choices parents unknowingly make today that increase the odds their child will be sick. My goal is to help you see both the choices that have a big impact and those that have lesser impacts because both work together to give our children the best chance at blossoming.

I will be honest: this isn't always easy. The medical system and our industries are set up to solve problems, not to prevent problems from happening. Doctors and drug companies will race to find treatments for a condition, but little value is placed on prevention. You also may struggle to stop the litany of "normal" things that are actually bad for your baby's health, especially unhealthy food, pollution, and chemical-laden products. But I'm here to help you as best I can.

As I battled to uncover what caused my son to become sick and then fought even harder to bring him closer to health, I realized that policy makers, doctors, and corporate leaders are people just like you and me. They, too, are parents who are raising sick children and they, too, want to see the threat of immune disease lifted. Which is why all change starts with individuals making better decisions with better information.

I was not able to prevent my child from developing eczema, food allergies, and asthma. But it's not all bad news in my house. Once I learned about the microbiome and began paying attention to the signals his microbiome was sending, we have slowly pulled medicine after medicine out of the cabinet. *Leo is no longer on any daily medications.* He technically still has ten food allergies and asthma, but he has not had a flare-up of his asthma in years, his skin is clear and does not itch, and his energy levels are that of a normal kid. His eyes are brighter, his sleep has improved, and his tantrums are rare because he feels better.

Bucking "normal" was not easy, and it required listening to what the clinical studies said, even when doctors we consulted didn't yet know the same information. But in the time that we changed our diets and our household habits and practices, we improved the entire family's health, making those of us who didn't exactly feel sick find a new level of healing.

Finally, as a lifelong believer and participant in the medical system, I find myself in a strange place regularly recommending "alternative" treatments to my friends. Yet year after year, more data is emerging to justify a precautionary principle toward what we allow in and on our bodies. More and more people are listening, and I believe that is slowly starting to change things. Paying attention is exactly how we get to a healthier place. One parent at a time, choosing a healthy life for their children.

Let's get started.

THE BABY
and
THE BIOME

CHAPTER ONE

The Rise of Immune Diseases

Common Misconception:
Food allergies are genetic.

Many people assume that food allergies are entirely hereditary, and that if there's no incidence of a food allergy anywhere in the family tree, a child will be fine. I used to believe this, too, and that's why I was floored when my son developed allergies that no one else on either side of the family had. The fact is that while some of the risk for food allergies does lie in a child's genetics, it's not like some babies have an allergy gene.[1] The real risk of developing food allergies rests in the food children eat, the medicines they take, the pathogens and environmental factors they face, and more.[2] By protecting against these things, a parent can protect their child's immune system from breaking down and triggering a massive allergic response.

When Scott and I took Leo home from the hospital after his asthma attack, we unpacked our bags with even more prescriptions than we'd had before. There were so many medicines that we couldn't find a drawer big enough to hold them, and we spread them out on his old changing table like a bootleg pharmacy.

Leo now had a daily antihistamine to prevent itching and skin flares and three different topical steroids to treat the flares that happened no matter what preventative measures we took. He had a daily inhaler to prevent asthma attacks and a rescue inhaler in case he had an attack anyway. These medications were on top of the special soaps, detergents, and emollients we already used. He was on a strict avoidance diet to prevent him from having an allergic reaction, but we also had three sets of EpiPens in case he accidentally ate one of those foods and had an allergic reaction anyway.

Have you noticed a pattern of futility yet?

I am not one to suffer—or parent—in silence, so as we settled into our new "normal," I began opening up to friends and family about the pain of watching my child hurt and my fears about his future. When I started talking with others, I thought I was the only one dealing with a sick kid, but I quickly discovered I was wrong. As Dr. Julia Getzelman, a pediatrician and functional medicine practitioner in San Francisco, said to me, "Today, doctors and parents spend a lot of time dealing with chronic noninfectious illnesses such as food allergy, eczema, asthma, autoimmunity, inflammatory bowel disease, celiac, and more. All of these conditions—many of which used to only plague adults—are now being considered normal in the pediatric population."

Every teacher I talked to saw multiple cases of one or the other in each class, and every pediatrician I encountered said each week they treated at least ten or twenty patients with these conditions. The more I looked, the more widespread immune diseases seemed to be, even among people I thought of as healthy.

What was going on?

....

What Are Allergic and Autoimmune Diseases?

The first thing you should know is that all allergic diseases (like the food allergies and eczema Leo suffers from) are actually immune diseases. Not all immune diseases are allergic diseases, though. For example, Type 1 diabetes, rheumatoid arthritis, and lupus do not develop because of allergic reactions. Some immune diseases are classified as *autoimmune diseases* and are distinct from allergic diseases for reasons I will describe below. Finally, all immune diseases—both allergic and autoimmune—are sometimes called *self-diseases* because they involve a normal body system going haywire.

Each immune disease affects a different part of the body: eczema happens in the skin, asthma in the lungs, celiac in the colon, food allergies in the gut, type 1 diabetes in the pancreas, and rheumatoid arthritis in the joints. While it is possible to have many immune diseases at once (like seemingly everyone I talked to), each condition is triggered by a different combination of genetics, environmental factors, or even viruses. But at its core, every manifestation of an immune disease is the same: the immune system malfunctions, goes rogue, and attacks something it shouldn't.

All allergic diseases are actually immune diseases. Not all immune diseases are allergic diseases, though.

I've used the term *flare* casually in my descriptions of Leo's illnesses, but the term deserves more explanation. A flare is a sudden intense onset of the symptoms of any immune disease brought on by a trigger. In the case of inflammatory bowel disease (IBD), a flare can mean intense cramping or diarrhea from eating spicy foods, drinking alcohol, or having too much sugar (all of which can be triggers). For Hashimoto's thyroiditis or lupus, it can mean fatigue or aches and pains caused by everything from gluten to stress to certain kinds of drugs. For asthma, it means significant difficulty breathing after a person is exposed to environmental allergens or, in Leo's case, a cold virus. These immune responses may come in waves, with days or weeks of flare-ups, and a person may have long periods of remission with no symptoms.

If the immune system attacks *internal* proteins or cells of the body that it should really leave alone, it's classified as an autoimmune disease. In the case of type 1 diabetes, the immune system goes after the beta cells that produce insulin. As the beta cells are killed off, the pancreas is destroyed, and the body is no longer able to produce insulin. Crohn's disease, ulcerative colitis, and IBD are all caused by a perpetual attack on the cells that make up the intestinal lining. This chronic inflammation of the digestive tract eventually destroys the intestines or colon.

Allergic diseases happen when the immune system attacks an *external* protein like pollen, food, or mold (antigens) that it should also ignore. The damage to the body is a side effect of an attack on the antigen, rather than from a direct attack on a healthy tissue. However, the immune response that occurs in an allergic response sometimes causes symptoms very similar to those we see in autoimmune diseases. Over time, if people experience a persistent allergic response like uncontrolled eczema, it can eventually destroy their tissue. All in all, the self-diseases we call immune disease are dangerous and, far too often, deadly.

Immune diseases can be hard for some people to wrap their brains around, so I find it helpful to think of them in terms of other, more tangible or familiar diseases. Think of the coronavirus that causes COVID-19. A person does not go to the hospital, get strapped to a ventilator, or die specifically because they contract this particular type of coronavirus or one of its many mutants. A person suffers through *the immune response to the coronavirus,* which may include shortness of breath, loss of taste and smell, fatigue, and unfortunately, sometimes organ failure leading to death. This cluster of immune responses is the disease called COVID-19.

Similarly, you are already familiar with another group of self-diseases: cancer. Consider three common cancers: breast, cervical, and lung. Breast cancer is triggered by genetics, cervical cancer by a virus (HPV), and lung cancer by pollutants that you breathe. In cancers, both internal (genes) and external (viruses or pollutants) root causes can make the normal body process of cell replication go haywire. In each cancer, cells replicate in a tissue incorrectly, and this malignant growth eventually harms an organ, causes sickness, or leads to death.

Cancer can sometimes be stopped by removing the root cause of the particular case (for example, think of quitting smoking), but often the disease is relentless and won't end without treatment. Luckily, allergic diseases can usually be stopped by removing the triggers. For example, if you're allergic to peanuts, you can avoid eating peanut butter. In autoimmune diseases, however, it can be impossible to remove the cell or protein the immune system is attacking, and without proper treatment, the disease may become relentless. As happens with cancer, the symptoms of allergic and autoimmune diseases may come and go despite your best efforts to manage them, and the true damage can be hard to see.

Because this book is about the emerging research on the conditions that my son has, most of what I discuss focuses on allergic disease. I will sometimes talk about allergic disease and sometimes about allergic and autoimmune disease when both apply. Just remember that all of them are diseases resulting from the malfunction of the immune system or, as I call them, *immune diseases.*

Finally, there is a huge overlap between the people who suffer from allergic disease and those who have autoimmune diseases. For example, children with type 1 diabetes are more likely to have asthma. Since these diseases often go hand in hand, I find it easiest to refer to them under a blanket term: *immune disease.*

Now let's try to make sense of this all.

....

The Immune System

To get this whole story across, we have to start at the top. The immune system is a mind-blowingly complex and effective system designed to keep you alive and your body healthy. As we go about our days, we are exposed to millions of different viruses, bacteria, molds, chemicals, heavy metals, and more from the air, surfaces, and food. All of these things can hurt us, and your immune system is always working to sort out the helpful stuff from the dangerous stuff, then clear the bad guys out—all without your noticing a thing.

You are born with part of your immune system—your *innate immunity.* This includes your barrier organs like the skin, gut, and lungs, and the cells that fight off bad stuff. Think of innate immunity as the infrastructure in an airport that keeps us safe: the security scanner, the police on Segways, and the computers that keep data on everyone going through the check-in counter and boarding gates. *Adaptive* or *acquired immunity,* on the other hand, develops as you go through the world and interact with things. This consists of the antibodies and other cells your body develops to become more efficient at recognizing threats and dealing with them.

A good analogy for the immune system is the brain. Babies are born with almost all the neurons they will ever have. These neurons are the intelligence infrastructure. But over time, these neurons shape and connect to one another to adapt to the world you encounter. The connections in your neurons create knowledge and memory, making your brain more efficient, too.

As I mentioned in the introduction, a child's immune development is timebound. In the first thousand days of their life—roughly three years, from newborn to toddlerhood—a child doubles, then triples, in size and learns to walk, talk, and socialize. While innate immunity is set from birth, the foundation for their adaptive immunity is formed during those first thousand days, with the first six months to a year being more critical and impactful than the second two years.

The outside influences a baby experiences play a critical role in how the immune system develops. Just as physical or emotional trauma in infancy can lead a brain to develop in unhelpful ways, environmental exposures in infancy can cause a person's immune system to develop in disease-prone ways as well.

> A child's immune development is timebound, with the first six months to a year being the most critical and impactful.

THE BARRIER ORGANS OF THE IMMUNE SYSTEM

The skin, gastrointestinal tract, and lungs are the largest immunologic organs in the body. All have an incredible amount of surface area that is constantly exposed to the outside environment, and they face the most common antigens—pollens, dander, dust, and foods—through the air, via contact with the skin, or through food when eating. Ideally, this large surface area should act as a stable barrier against pathogens.

As food, water, and anything else passes through the long unbroken tube that extends from the opening of your mouth through to your stomach and the intestines and eventually to your anus, some things are selectively allowed to cross the barrier and enter your body. The rest is flushed out. When you walk outside and face pollution, pathogens, and other environmental factors, your skin also acts like a barricade, allowing some things in and blocking others. Your lungs are not a tube, but a balloon, with your mouth and nose representing the open end. As with food, air is allowed into the balloon. Your body selectively allows oxygen into your bloodstream and then pushes everything else back out when you exhale.

Together, your skin, your gastrointestinal tract, and your lungs make up the barrier that protects you from the outside world. These barriers are also called your *epithelium,* and the cells of all the barriers are called *epithelial cells.* The skin is made of multiple layers of epithelial cells and is covered in proteins like ceramides. The gut barrier has a thick mucus that coats the epithelial cells and protects them from the acidic environment. The lungs are covered with a mucus as well—something you most often notice when you have a chest cold.

Different parts of the epithelial barrier contain their own mechanisms for immune defenses, in fact. For example, the intestines can distinguish between foreign pathogens and safe nutrient proteins. The esophagus and mouth each have their own systems that are attuned to proteins and bacteria, respectively, and the skin's defense mechanism is sensitive to parasites and chemicals. Finally, the lungs' immune system is particularly attentive to particles of different sizes.

If your epithelial barrier is dysfunctional or broken, however, outside things will get inside when they shouldn't. Your immune system is *designed* to react and continue to react until the invader is gone. And in general, your immune system is biased toward overreacting because the consequences of underreacting can be really, really bad. In the next section I'll try to explain how the immune cells react when things break or sneak through the barrier.

If your epithelial barrier is broken, outside things will get inside when they shouldn't.

THE CELLS OF THE IMMUNE SYSTEM

When you go to the airport to board a flight, one of your first steps is to stand in line so you can check in. This act ensures that you are allowed to fly and provides you with a boarding pass telling you which gate to go to at what time. You then line up at security with your boarding pass and identification so officials can make sure that you aren't carrying anything illegal or unsafe. The final step before you board involves your lining up (once again) at the gate so that the flight attendants can do one more verification. It's a long and often irritating process, but for the most part it's orderly and ensures that nothing and no one dangerous can get on a plane.

Now imagine how impossible security would be if thousands of people simultaneously entered the airport from the doors, windows, sewers, and loading docks, skipped security, and then ran to a random boarding gate. It would be a disaster.

Yet your immune system is basically running this very chaotic airport, trying to get nutrients and cells to the right places at the right time, all while weeding out any threats! It takes something close to magic to pull this off, but your immune system does it day in and day out.

The body does this with immune teams that are specialized into units, each with a specific assignment. Team 1 and Team 17 (aka Th1 and Th17) are designed to react to bacteria and viruses. These teams can sense bacteria and viruses that shouldn't be in your body or cells that have been infected by a virus or bacterium. Teams 1 and 17 use their friends, killer T cells, which are always roving around in your blood, to destroy cells that have been infected and keep the bacterium or virus from replicating. Team 1 and Team 17 can also flood your body with mucus to dislodge and flush bacteria out.

Team 1 and Team 17 create tags, usually IgG antibodies, to latch on to bacteria or viruses so that the killer cells know where to go. The super cool thing is that once you have these tags, or antibodies, they stick around and float around. The next time the same bacterium or virus tries to show up at the airport, it is immediately identified and booted out quietly. In many cases, your body will keep this memory forever, making you immune to attack from those specific bacteria or viruses.

The next team you need to know about is Team 2 (aka Th2). It specializes in dealing with parasites. Team 2 uses different innate immune cells to do its work, including B cells, mast cells, and eosinophils. These cells live in various tissues throughout your body, including the gut, nose, and lung mucus. Team 2 also has its own set of flags to become more efficient over time; these are called IgE antibodies.

Team 2 cells fight parasites by releasing a massive amount of histamine, which can cause vomiting, diarrhea, tightness in the airways, a drop in blood pressure, horrible itching, sneezing, and in the worst cases, shock and death, depending on where it is released. All of these symptoms work effectively to kill or expel parasites.

(Side note: Very recently, researchers have found that IgA antibodies and other mysterious signals can also tell the body to fight parasites in the intestinal tract by causing an inflammation of the lining, perhaps in an effort to dislodge parasites. This inflammation has been termed a lot of things, including the diseases enterocolitis syndrome (FPIES), proctocolitis, eosinophilic esophagitis (EoE), and more. These illnesses feel very similar to the gut inflammation of autoimmune diseases like Crohn's disease. But they are technically allergies triggered by certain foods, and symptoms can stop when people remove that food from their diet.)

Team 2 is responsible for a whole range of allergies, including eczema, food allergies, asthma, hay fever, food-protein-induced FPIES, EoE, and more. To say it again, each of these diseases is the result of the same dysfunction—a Th2 response to an antigen—but they are simply expressed in different ways and in different organs.*

The last immune team you need to meet is the Regulatory Team (aka Treg). This team is the body's defense against mucous floods or histamine releases getting out of hand. It is always riding around the body, policing the other immune teams. After all, your immune system wants to get rid of bad guys, but it wants you to stay healthy while it does. Your Regulatory Team (using Treg, Breg, NKreg, and other cells) should prevent an overreaction, but sometimes it doesn't. That problem occurs when the regulatory cells are missing or if there is a barrier dysfunction, which weakens them and makes them stand down.

---

* Every year we are uncovering more about how this all works. Recently T follicular helper cells were also found to be important for allergies. I don't discuss them here because the science is still new.

HOW IMMUNE DISEASES HAPPEN

If we zoom out to think about the cellular immune system and epithelial barrier organs together, it's clear that the singular purpose of the immune system is to protect you from dangerous things in the outside world getting into you and staying there. As Dr. Christine Olsen, the founder of the Broad Institute's Food Allergy Science Initiative (a joint project of MIT and Harvard), said to me, "The immune system is your body's quality control system."

The immune system is great when it correctly fights off things that would otherwise harm us. Immune *diseases* happen when the immune system messes up and attacks something that isn't actually a virus, bacterium, or parasite. An allergy is when Team 2 sees and mislabels a pollen as a parasite and attacks it. An autoimmune disease is when Team 1 or Team 17 accidentally believes your own cells are part of a bacterial or viral threat and assaults them day after day.

As a reminder: your immune system has a built-in mechanism to stop the immune teams from making mistakes, which is the Regulatory Team. One of the fundamental differences between people with immune diseases and those without is that they have too few regulatory cells telling the immune system to take it easy. For example, when you get sick with a cold, Treg cells are important to keep your immune response from spinning out of control.

We really need the Regulatory Teams to prevent mistakes because once a team has messed up and decided a safe thing (pollen or your own tissue) is dangerous, the only way to stop the immune attack is to remove the antigen or smother the immune cells with medicines. For instance, allergic reactions can be prevented by avoiding triggering foods and pollens or treating the symptoms with antihistamines. Autoimmune diseases can some-times be stopped by removing the tissue the body is attacking, such as when Crohn's patients choose to undergo a surgery that removes part of their intestines. But if getting rid of the trigger or tissue doesn't work, the only other option many people have to alleviate their painful symptoms is to take daily steroids and biologics, each of which smothers the immune system attack.

With my son, his allergies occur because his Team 2 over-reacts to things it perceives as threats. The prescriptions (steroids, inhalers, EpiPens) all work by shutting down or smothering the response. But none of them address the root issues: that his Team 2 cells are overactive and that he doesn't have a strong enough Regulatory Team to calm them back down.

Unfortunately, Leo is far from alone. Until the 1990s, almost everyone's immune systems operated their entire life without making a mistake. Today, 10 percent of children have IgE food allergies to peanuts, wheat, tree nuts, eggs, dairy, and soy.[3] Per-haps a much larger group have non-IgE allergies.[4] (I talk more about IgE and non-IgE food allergies in chapter 4.) More and more adolescents and adults are developing food and environ-mental allergies, meaning that their immune systems are sud-denly attacking antigens the person tolerated for years. More people are developing more than one allergy, and others are experiencing increasingly bad symptoms of those allergies. This suggests that their immune teams are getting more trigger-happy or their Regulatory Teams are falling down on the job.

Science shows us that our environment and how we treat our bodies plays a clear role in how our immune systems react. What is it in particular about our environment, diet, medication use, habits, and more, though?

Today, 10 percent of children have IgE food allergies to peanuts, wheat, tree nuts, eggs, dairy, and soy.

What are we as a society doing to cause such harm to our kids? Because the data is clear: immune diseases are everywhere, and their incidence is growing.

Before we move on, let's recap a few key points because they will come up again.

1. The immune system has different teams to deal with different types of threats. Broadly speaking, Team 1 (Th1) is for viruses, Team 2 (Th2) is for parasites, and Team 17 (Th17) is for bacteria.
2. The immune system fights bad guys (viruses, parasites, and bacteria) by creating memory files, or antibodies, specific to each one. Usually these memories are permanent.
3. Allergic and autoimmune diseases can happen only when immune teams make the mistake of identifying something harmless as dangerous. No one is born with these mistakes.
4. The Regulatory Team is a critical part of keeping the immune system in balance. When regulatory cells aren't doing their job of stopping an overreaction, allergic and autoimmune diseases become more likely.

IMMUNE DISEASES ARE AN EPIDEMIC

My grandmother was born in India before World War I. She had nine children over twenty years, but she and my grandfather buried five of them in childhood. My father was told that as a result of an unpaid debt, a ghost haunted their house and that any children born within those walls were taken as repayment. I suspect my grandparents made up that story because it was the best explanation they had at the time—or at least the one that would make the most sense to young children, even if it terrified them. The truth was, though, that the two children closest in age to my father, including his beloved sister, died from a typhoid outbreak that he somehow survived.

By the time millennials like me were born in the United States, losing a child to a pathogen was practically unthinkable. Polio had gone from an annual summer stalker to a distant memory. Barring the occasional cluster in areas with low vaccination rates, measles, mumps, and rubella were eradicated decades ago,[5] and the same is true for diphtheria, tetanus, and tuberculosis. Smallpox—the most terrifying disease in human history, which decimated Native American empires—was so thoroughly wiped out that we stopped vaccinating against it. The COVID-19 pandemic has made us aware that we aren't free from the specter of pathogens, but the fact that young children have fallen ill and died at such low rates has provided families a small degree of comfort.

Just as we were settled into the twentieth century and had begun to feel confident that we'd claimed victory against pathogenic diseases, a switch flipped. Sometime between 1985 and 1995, a new epidemic began to spread, eventually affecting the same percentage of children as the vanquished diseases did in the past. But this time, the enemy was our own bodies. Our new self-diseases are in many ways more insidious than the pathogens that used to terrify us. In the same way that my grandmother's generation expected to lose half of their children to a virus or infection, today we expect that 40 to 50 percent of children will develop immune disease.[6]

Let's put that into perspective. Philadelphia's Pennsylvania Hospital—the nation's oldest hospital and where my two boys were born—performs over 5,000 deliveries each year. By the time those 5,000 babies reach preschool, at least 20 percent, or 1,000, will require special care to handle their eczema, food allergies, or asthma. Each of these conditions requires daily medication and management that limits what activities they can participate in, where they can go, and what they can eat. By kindergarten, an additional 500 of those children will have added seasonal allergies into the mix. The school nurse's drawers will be stocked with EpiPens, albuterol rescue inhalers, and over-the-counter antihistamines.

Both autism and attention deficit hyperactivity disorder (ADHD) are increasingly being defined as immune diseases and can exist on a spectrum from manageable to debilitating. When kindergarten starts, perhaps 100 of the babies will require specialized instruction for their autism, and up to 1,000 will be on prescription medication for ADHD.

By the time they reach college, more severe autoimmune diseases will have developed in 300 children. The National Institutes of Health (NIH) estimates that 5 to 8 percent of Americans have a severe autoimmune disease. This category includes type 1 diabetes, rheumatoid arthritis, lupus, psoriasis, celiac disease, Hashimoto's thyroiditis, inflammatory bowel diseases including Crohn's and ulcerative colitis, and multiple sclerosis. Autoimmune diseases are being diagnosed in people of all ages and walks of life, slowly eating away at critical body systems like the intestines, pancreas, or thyroid. While the symptoms of autoimmune disease can be mitigated, the overall effect is debilitating and worsens with time.

Because most immune sufferers are affected by multiple conditions, the exact numbers are hard to estimate. However, it would be a lowball to estimate that 2,000 (40 percent) of those perfect Pennsylvania Hospital babies will enter adulthood restricted from traveling, attending the university of their choice, or holding down a job where exposures to triggers cannot be avoided.

It gets worse. Look up any of the immune diseases mentioned

above, and you will find a specialist in that field using the word *epidemic* to describe what they are seeing. Prevalence rates of each disease—meaning the number of people who have a particular condition—have doubled and maybe tripled in the last thirty years alone. And it's not stopping. We seem to be developing new conditions every decade. Meat allergy, or alpha-gal allergy, was identified less than ten years ago, but already cases have been found in nearly every part of the country.[7]

....

The Search for Answers

I previously drew a comparison between immune disease and the other big self-disease, cancer. Another way that immune diseases are like cancer is that when cancer was first discovered, all the efforts of the scientific and medical establishment went into stopping its progress. We developed ways to cut out tumors, shrink them with radiation, or stop the growth of cancer cells with chemotherapy. Only much later did we ask *why* people were developing cancer, how we could prevent it, and begin taking precautionary steps like trying to remove carcinogens from our environment.

As cases of immune disease have risen dramatically over the last thirty to forty years, almost everyone—from doctors to parents to educators—has focused on how to stop them after they happen. We have created artificial insulin, shut off immune cells (with steroids and biologics), and reduced flares with immunotherapy. But only recently, in the past decade, have people really started to dig into *why* immune diseases are developing at such a drastic pace.

Overdiagnosis is a tempting and yet insufficient explanation for our current state. We have known about food allergies and rhinitis for over a hundred years, so there's no reason doctors would suddenly start diagnosing those conditions only thirty years ago. With symptoms including swelling, low blood pressure, rapid pulse, and vomiting, anaphylaxis—which can be deadly—is impossible to fake. Yet ER visits for anaphylaxis have doubled every five years from the mid-1990s.[8] There's no such thing as phony asthma, either; just ask the nurse who admitted Leo to the hospital. She might tell you that asthma rates have gone up across all sex, racial, and ethnic groups since the early 1980s. Finally, the Centers for Disease Control and Prevention (CDC) reported in early 2020 that type 1, or juvenile, diabetes increased 30 percent in the United States between 2002 and 2015.[9] Unmanaged diabetes is fatal, so there is almost no chance that people lived with it undiagnosed before.

Genetics also cannot explain the rise in immune disease. First and foremost, genes don't change within a generation. Lactase persistence, or the ability to digest lactase protein in cow's milk, took somewhere between 50 and 150 generations to become common in Europeans.[10] Almost every increase in allergic and autoimmune diseases has happened in about one generation. Even epigenetics, the idea that external influences affect our DNA, doesn't explain enough, because we would notice trends that children in the same family develop the same diseases. We know that babies missing a gene to code the protein filaggrin are more likely to develop eczema. But the gene for filaggrin didn't suddenly go missing in the last thirty years.

Most recently, there have been several studies in respected medical journals hypothesizing that immune diseases are caused by the lack of exposure to bacteria and viruses (called the hygiene hypothesis[11]) and the lack of exposure to parasites (called the helminth hypothesis[12]). Unfortunately, additional studies have failed to find a clear link between these two distinct issues and immune disease. Some studies have even shown that avoiding viruses in infancy can prevent immune disease.

....

Where We Have Arrived

When my son was faced with a lifetime of taking medicine and I watched my vision of his future start to fade, I wanted answers.

Thanks to research in the last few years, it turns out there *is* an underlying explanation for our out-of-control immune diseases. What scientists are showing is that our immune cells and our barriers seem to be malfunctioning simultaneously.[13]

Babies born today enter a world that is unlike anything humans have seen before. Their skin and lungs are bombarded daily with chemical stressors that didn't exist thirty years ago, and their guts are dealing with a brand-new diet. What's more, the strength of your child's skin, lungs, and gut relies on a complex interaction between them and the bacteria, fungi, and other microbes that live on these barriers. I'll explain in the next chapter how exactly this relationship works. For now, know that two decades ago, we barely understood that we are covered in bacteria and that they make up a significant portion of our immune system. Today, we know that we cannot appreciate the true problem of immune disease without first understanding our microbiome.

> **There *is* an underlying explanation for our out-of-control immune diseases. What scientists are showing is that our immune cells and our barriers seem to be malfunctioning simultaneously.**

CHAPTER TWO

....

Meet Your Real Baby

Common Misconception:
In the human microbiome, there are
"good" and "bad" microbes.

....

While there are some microbes that are simply bad news, most can be both good and bad. It all depends on where they are in or on your body and what other microbes are around them. The bacterium *Staphylococcus epidermidis* is critical for healthy skin, but if it gets into your bloodstream from a cut or medical procedure, it can cause a deadly illness. Similarly, *Staphylococcus aureus* is normal on your skin. But if *S. aureus* is too abundant or if the presence of *S. epidermidis* does not keep it in check, it will basically punch holes in your skin, which breaks the barrier. *Escherichia coli* is another great example. If certain strains of *E. coli* are ingested through contaminated water, milk, produce, or meat, they can cause diarrhea. If they enter the urethra (by sex or poor hygiene), you can develop urinary tract infections. However,

E. coli is not all bad. This bacterium occurs naturally in the gut, and it helps break down the food you eat and triggers your body to create more Treg cells, which may help prevent immune disease.

The earliest research into the microbiome was carried out in the 1680s, when a Dutch merchant decided to compare a stool sample and a saliva sample under his microscope. He remarked how different the microbes swimming under the glass looked, but he didn't stop to think about their profound effects on human health.

For hundreds of years, doctors and scientists did much the same. They knew about the existence of the microscopic universe of bacteria, fungi, parasites, and viruses that are in and on us, and they knew that this environment differs based on where in the body these microbes live. But they believed the microbiome was a strange artifact of our hunter-gatherer days, that it did next to nothing for us, and that it could be removed without noticeably or negatively changing our health. They also understood that—at their worst—our microbes were a nuisance and sometimes harmful. For example, nurses and doctors scrub a patient's skin before surgery because the bacteria on the skin can cause infections if they get inside an incision. You wash your face at night because the microbes in your pores can cause acne, and you change out of sweaty socks not just because they're uncomfortable, but because the fungus on your toes can cause athlete's foot.

Only since the late 2000s have we *truly* begun to wrap our brains around the microbiome's role in our bodies, and today we understand that it certainly isn't entirely harmful. It's also much more complicated than the probiotics aisle at Whole Foods may lead you to believe.

The microbiome is *who we are.*

....

Microbes Make Us Who We Are

For hundreds of years, we have thought of ourselves as a singular creature, built from our own DNA. I majored in engineering in college and took my fair share of biology classes, but my assumption about our physical and chemical makeup was still just as naive. I knew that each of us contains diverse colonies of microbes all over and inside our bodies, but the microbiome didn't hold much mystery or allure to me. Like the appendix, I thought, it was just *there.*

How wrong I was. How wrong we *all* were.[1] Scientific advances of the last fifteen years, particularly in rapid genetic sequencing, have unveiled that we are actually only 1 percent human by gene count. The human genome provides about 20,000 genes, while the microbiome is estimated to contain about 2 million, or 99 percent, of our genes. We are microbe storage machines.

> The human genome provides about 20,000 genes, while the microbiome is estimated to contain about 2 million, or 99 percent, of our genes.

As is true of an apartment building in Manhattan, filled to the brim with families, you can get good renters who will replace facades, repair damage, and make lovely roof gardens. Or you can get bad renters who will destroy floors and leave out food that draws roaches and rodents into the walls. It may be hard from afar to tell the good ones from the bad ones, but a building filled with conscientious dwellers will last hundreds of years, while a building with noxious dwellers can be quickly destroyed.

The Human Microbiome Project—which was launched in 2007 to sequence the genes of the microbes living on 250 healthy adults—has documented more than 10,000 different microbial species living on or in humans.[2] The gut has about 1,000 species, while the mouth has an additional 300, the skin 850, and the urogenital tract another 1,000. This does not count the fungi, viruses, and parasites that are also included in the balance. One square inch of our skin can have up to 6 billion microorganisms living on it, and the average adult has 3,000 square inches of skin.

Yet most people are rightfully terrified of microbes. Malaria (a parasite of the genus *Plasmodium*) has killed at least 10 percent of humans throughout history. The Justinian plague (bacterium *Yersinia pestis*) may have wiped out 50 percent of the people that were alive in AD 540.[3] Possibly 90 percent of Native Americans were killed not in fighting but by diseases brought from Europe (smallpox, measles, and flu).[4] Thousands of years of watching our loved ones die from microbes told us one thing: we cannot live with them.

However, after spending the nineteenth and twentieth centuries removing microbes from our bodies with antibiotics, pasteurization, pesticides, disinfectants, antibacterial soaps, and hand sanitizer, we have also learned that we cannot live *without* them.

Why? Since scientists realized that every crevice of our bodies is teeming with microbes, they also discovered that most of what we thought were bodily functions are actually microbial functions. The nutrients and vitamins you need and use from food are actually pulled out by bacteria that live in your intestines. The protective oils that keep your skin healthy are not produced by your skin cells, but by the microbes that live on your

> Much of our immune system is in constant communication with our microbiome. Our microbes can actually turn our immune cells on or off.

skin. And critically to the topic of immune disease, much of our immune system is in constant communication with our microbiome. Our microbes can actually turn our immune cells on or off, keeping us either in good balance or plagued by disease.

What are all these microbes doing riding around in us? Microbes exist in three ways in nature, and thus there are three types of relationships we have with the microbes in our microbiomes.

OUR BODY'S RELATIONSHIP WITH MICROBES[5]

The first kind of microbe, which you've no doubt heard of, are parasites. Parasites feed off their host and hurt that host when it is advantageous for them. In this context I'm not talking about the larger multicellular organisms like ticks and head lice. I mean the microbes that exist in our microbiome, including *Plasmodium* (the malaria bug). This category was the first to be identified by scientists and the one we spent the nineteenth century eradicating through pasteurization, clean water programs, improved public health, better sewage systems, and more.

Second are commensal microbes, or ones indifferent to us and merely along for the ride. *Staphylococcus aureus,* which is found in many people's noses, may fall into this category because it seems to serve no purpose. *Helicobacter pylori,* a bacterium that survives in almost every person's extremely acidic stomach, is another commensal microbe.

Third are mutually beneficial microbes, which help us complete a function while we help them survive as well. There are bacteria in the intestine that feed off undigested fibers in our food and cannot get this fiber without us. They then excrete certain nutrients that we are unable to extract ourselves from food. We benefit from them, and they benefit from us.

As we learn more about the microbiome, these categorizations are constantly changing. For example, *H. pylori* was found to cause stomach ulcers and stomach cancers, which would classify it as a harmful parasite. But its presence also prevents gastric reflux and esophageal damage, making it appear to be mutually beneficial. Hookworms, a parasite that can cause abdominal pain, diarrhea, weight loss, and anemia in severe cases, may also signal our immune system to calm down, thus preventing allergic disease. Does that mean a hookworm isn't a harmful parasite and instead can be considered commensal? Yes, sort of, if you feel you must categorize these things.

In general, no matter which relationship type the microbes have with your body, they are simply trying to survive. They are happy to be living where they are, so they utilize different mechanisms to stop other microbes from taking their territory. Sometimes they even work with other microbes to thrive together.

Some microbes in our microbiome share genes with our genome to get us to produce proteins that enhance their food or to kill off their enemies. Microbes may hijack or participate in our immune system, utilizing it to kill competition or turning it off to allow themselves to thrive. Microbes even drive our behaviors, sending signals through our nervous system to create food cravings so that we will eat the food they prefer!

In short, we owe much of our biology and our individuality to microbes that live on and in our bodies.

The way our microbes use us may sound nefarious, but it all depends on how you look at it. The best way to think of our microbiome, and us, is as part of an ecosystem. Most creatures in an ecosystem are both predator and prey, which means that most provide benefits to some species and harm to others. A balance between all the competing interests is necessary for any ecosystem to thrive.

We have many ecosystems within the planet that is our body. The microbiome of each location is unique depending on how much light, oxygen, warmth, acidity, oil, and food it gets. Some species make up billions of organisms in one section of the body, while other species may have only a hundred members in their group. These are sometimes called *keystone species,* which are rare but critical to the proper functioning of the ecosystem. For example, the bacterium *Ruminococcus bromii,* which exists in the colon, has the special ability to break down certain starches that other bacteria who greatly outnumber it cannot.

A healthy ecosystem—both in the wild and in your body—depends on the total count of organisms, their diversity of species, and the presence of specific species. If we eradicate *Ruminococcus bromii,* for example, the colon won't digest starch properly. In *The Lion King,* a movie I loved as a child, Mufasa tells his son, Simba that all the animals in their kingdom exist in a balance. Simba, must respect every creature from every species in that balance, not just the ones he sees. When Mufasa was killed, Simba's uncle, Scar, banished him and took over the throne. Scar then immediately overhunted the antelope. Eventually the entire ecosystem broke down, and the hyenas had a ball.

A microbiome out of balance or with the wrong mix of species for us to thrive is called a *dysbiotic microbiome,* and it can be just as chaotic as a party full of wild predators. It is a microbial ecosystem that is not functioning to keep its host and itself healthy. That host could be you, your aging parents, or, in the case of this book, your baby.

We like to separate things into good and bad, but microbiomes are not really either. There isn't a "correct" microbiome. A wide variety of possible combinations of microbes are workable, and an equal number of combinations are dysbiotic. Dysbiosis (the condition of having a dysbiotic microbiome) can come from a missing keystone species, too few microbes overall, or too little diversity in the microbial species. For the rest of this book, I will use the term *dysbiosis* to mean a microbiome that is causing or allowing an allergic or autoimmune disease.

> **Dysbiosis (the condition of having a dysbiotic microbiome) can come from a missing keystone species, too few microbes overall, or too little diversity in the microbial species.**

MEET THE MICROBIOME OF THE SKIN[6]

The skin is a human's largest organ, and the cells that make it up serve as a first line of defense against many potential invaders. The skin is also the organ that interacts the most with the outside world, including clothing, chemicals, soaps, air pollution, and pathogens. The skin is colonized by the same bacteria, fungi, viruses, and mites found in one's environment, and it is constantly in flux as the environment changes. Some microbes that populate the skin can be harmful, like *S. aureus,* which can cause everything from skin infections to pneumonia, toxic shock syndrome, and sepsis. Others can be helpful and play a role in educating the immune memory cells to recognize antigens.

Babies are thought to get their starter skin microbiome from the vaginal canal and then from skin-to-skin contact with their mother right after birth. From that point on, as a baby interacts with clothing materials, the dust and dander in its household, and the dirt and grass in the local park, the species that make up the skin microbiome change.

The skin's microbiome is incredibly diverse, and it will differ from one body part to another depending on the environmental demands it faces and that section's natural oil levels. The skin on your hands has a microbiome that differs from the skin under your arms, for example. The physical and chemical features of skin in different parts of the body select for different sets of microbes that are best adapted to that environment. In general, the skin is cool, acidic, and dry, but its microenvironments form based on skin thickness, folds, the number of hair follicles, and the presence of glands.[7] We are just starting to identify and understand the viruses and fungi that live on skin, and they are likely an important part of the ecosystem as well.

The microbes on your skin help create and enhance its strength. The outermost layer of the skin, the stratum corneum, consists of dead cells and lipids, which act like the bricks and mortar that form buildings. Together, they make up the epithelial barrier, which prevents pathogens from getting in and water from getting out.

As a first line of defense, the skin barrier is a vital part of the immune system. On an ongoing basis the immune system modulates the microbes on the skin, and the microbes on the skin do the same for the immune system. Receptors in the skin cells are designed to recognize pathogens by their surface proteins and chemicals, and they constantly check which microbes are colonizing the skin surface. When receptors spot a pathogen, they trigger an immune system response that directly kills pathogenic bacteria, fungi, and viruses.[8]

In the other direction, *Staphylococcus epidermidis* (a commensal bacterium) can activate the immune system to kill "bad" bacteria like *S. aureus* and group A strep via the immune receptors. *S. epidermidis* can also excrete an acid to the skin receptors that tells the immune system to turn down and limits skin inflammation.

Dysbiosis of the Skin[9]

I remember the first time I noticed Leo's eczema. He was only five months old, and I had taken him to London to visit my sister, her husband, and their kids. During a nap, when he was lying next to his cousins, I noticed that his cheeks seemed red in comparison to the girls' cheeks. I assumed that it was caused by the dry air from the airplane. The next day, however, my sister and I took our kids to a baby spa—mostly as a joke—and the owner made a remark about how dry Leo's skin was.

I didn't realize it at the time, but Leo was developing the classic signs of eczema. Eczema is a chronic inflammatory skin disease in which the outer layer of the skin becomes broken due to a loss of lipids (the mortar between skin cells, which holds them together like bricks). As I mentioned earlier, when the skin barrier is cracked, the immune system will spring into action against things that touch the skin and will stay on high alert until the surrounding landscape is "safe" again. The raw, inflamed, sometimes blistery skin characteristic of eczema is proof of that battle.

Dysbiosis of the skin microbiome can cause a breakdown of the skin barrier, allowing pollens, food dust, bacteria, or viruses to cross the skin barrier. These failures can eventually lead to psoriasis (raised patches of dry, itchy, or scaly skin), eczema, and contact dermatitis (a burning, itchy rash caused by contact with a foreign substance). In one example, free fatty acids of a particular length—which are excreted by *Cutibacterium* and *Corynebacterium* species—are crucial for the skin barrier, and if your baby is missing these species, their skin barrier can break down.

Patients with eczema are much more likely to carry *S. aureus* on their skin than are healthy people.[10] The amount of *S. aureus* on eczema patients also varies depending on its location. If you have a lesion—an actual hole in the skin barrier—you are much more likely to have significant amounts of *S. aureus* there. Eczema skin also shows much less microbial diversity than healthy skin and reduced numbers of certain kinds of bacteria, meaning *S. aureus* crowds out other—potentially good—bacteria.

> Dysbiosis of the skin microbiome can cause a breakdown of the skin barrier, allowing pollens, food dust, bacteria, or viruses to cross the skin barrier.

The microbiome doesn't always act alone. Filaggrin, a protein that helps bind epithelial cells, is a crucial component of the skin barrier, and people with a genetic mutation that causes filaggrin deficiency are more likely to have eczema. *S. aureus* attaches strongly to skin that's deficient in filaggrin, then increases the pH while reducing the ceramide levels. (Ceramides are fatty acids, or lipids, that make skin springy and keep it from cracking.)

Here's an example of how dysbiosis can cause things to spin out of control. If the bacterium *S. epidermis* isn't present in sufficient quantities to keep *S. aureus* in check, *S. aureus* creates a biofilm and releases a toxin into the skin. This toxin triggers the immune system to let out a chemical that causes a strong itch response.[11] What happens when you scratch an itch? You cause micro-tears in the skin, making your immune system go into higher alert.

Researchers have demonstrated that infants with eczema are more likely to develop peanut allergy if they have an *S. aureus* infection.[12] These babies have cracks in their skin barrier caused by both *S. aureus* and by scratching. Those breaks allow peanut dust from their parents' hands or from the carpet to penetrate the skin. When the immune system sees the innocent peanut in the same place as all this damage, Team 2 flags the peanut with IgE antibodies, causing allergic sensitization. Even worse, the act of scratching itchy skin and the high alert mode from the immune system trigger the development of more mast cells, which releases more histamine and provokes an anaphylactic allergic response.[13]

In short, dysbiosis of the skin can have far-reaching consequences—from eczema to food allergies to an extreme allergic reaction that may cause death.

Infants with eczema are more likely to develop peanut allergy if they have an *S. aureus* infection.

Moving past bacteria, the fungus *Malassezia* spp. lives largely on the face near the neck crease and may make up 80 percent of all skin fungi.[14] When a baby has cradle cap, or seborrheic dermatitis, is it thought to be from an overpopulation of *Malassezia* spp. on the scalp.[15] *Malassezia* eats sebum and releases oleic acid, which causes excessive skin cell shedding and inflammation. This is why anti-dandruff shampoos can reduce cradle cap, whereas antibacterials—which don't eradicate fungus like most dandruff shampoos do—have little effect.

The combination of certain *Malassezia* fungi with bacterial changes can worsen eczema. Eczema is much more severe in patients with *Malassezia globosa,* whereas people with more *Malassezia restricta* have mild eczema. This difference may be why even though cradle cap does not cause eczema, it often appears as a warning sign of future eczema.

We have not yet defined the remainder of skin fungi, but we do know that *Candida* spp. colonizes skin and can cause infection in people with immune deficiency, diabetes, or infection following antibiotics. Certain mites (such as *Demodex folliculorum* and *Demodex brevis*), which are small arthropods, are associated with rosacea as well as other skin disorders, including facial itching.

MEET THE MICROBIOME OF THE GUT

Your intestinal tract, usually called the gut, is where most of the microbes in your body live. As mentioned earlier, the GI tract is a big tube that goes through your body. Adding up its surface area, it's actually a bigger barrier than your skin. The GI tract barrier is particularly attuned to the kinds of things that try to get into your system through your food and water, like parasites.

The first stop for things in your intestinal tract is the mouth, which harbors over 700 species of bacteria.[16] Your mouth has microbes covering the teeth, the tongue, the cheeks, and the palate, and huge amounts of bacteria live right between the teeth and the gums. If you've ever gone to the dentist—and I hope that's all of you—you know that the bacteria on your teeth develop into plaque, and a dentist scrapes it away during a cleaning. The oral microbiome usually exists in the form of a biofilm, which is a giant community of microorganisms that sticks together and adheres to a surface (again, think of plaque). It plays a crucial role in early digestion, protecting the mouth from infection and preventing pathogens from making it further through the gut.

The oral microbiome is also constantly in flux. It changes each time you brush your teeth and every night when you go to sleep (when the oxygen levels in your mouth fluctuate). Because of the sensitivity to oxygen, the oral microbiomes of mouth breathers and closed-mouth nose breathers are different. And this difference may be why mouth breathers are much more prone to getting sick.

The next stop in the intestinal tract is the esophagus, which has a microbiome pretty similar to the mouth.[17] In a healthy esophagus, most of the bacteria are Gram-positive (meaning they can easily be killed by antibiotics), with a diverse number of species.

Your stomach is next, and it breaks down food, produces hormones, and fights infection via the immune cells that are present in its walls. Because the stomach is so acidic and is constantly compressing and squishing, scientists used to assume that nothing could live in it. It took until 1984 before scientists discovered that *H. pylori* could excrete ammonia, neutralize stomach acid, and embed itself in the mucous layer of the stomach.

From the stomach, food moves to the small intestine, where it is broken down into nutrients that are absorbed into the body. The small and large intestine have the highest concentration of bacteria, with up to 1,000 bacteria per gram in the large intestine.

The stomach passes all the indigestible fiber to the intestines, and it's here that super-critical bacteria break down that fiber to produce vitamin K, digest lactose, make essential amino acids, and carry out the transformation of bile. These microbes secrete small molecules that your body uses to regulate blood pressure. Intestinal bacteria also produce antimicrobial compounds and support the gut lining, preventing pathogens that have made it this far from attaching or breaking through.

The microbes of the intestine have a huge effect on your immune system.[18] Because most pathogens enter the body through the gut and the intestines are the site of nutrient absorption, the intestinal lining is a key interface between the immune system and the environment. Bacteria not only make most of the mucus that lines the intestine but also signal the immune system through receptors to recognize and attack specific pathogens.

The gut and the brain are incredibly connected, since they are both systems critical to our survival, and their interplay is called the *gut-brain axis*. The gut uses the brain or nervous system to recruit more immune cells and to push food back up (as vomit) or through the intestines and colon (as feces). The brain can use our gut to make us feel the "gut punch" of sadness, to suppress hunger when we need to focus, or to speed and slow digestion when we require it.

Given this cross talk, you may not be surprised that the microbiome of the intestine turns out to have an effect on your brain function and emotions. Gut bacteria have been implicated in mood disorders like depression, and the gut of early infancy is now thought to affect brain development, potentially causing ADHD and autism. It was also recently shown that babies who spend time in neonatal intensive care units can develop dysbiotic guts, sometimes resulting in lifelong brain damage.

> **The microbiome of the intestine turns out to have an effect on your brain function and emotions. The gut of early infancy is now thought to affect brain development, potentially causing ADHD and autism.**

The last stop in the digestive tract is the colon. The microbes in the colon use nondigestible carbohydrates like cellulose, oligosaccharides, and unabsorbed sugars and alcohols to produce short-chain fatty acids, thus aiding in food metabolism, extracting up to 15 percent of the calories that feed you.

How You Get Your Gut Biome

In utero, up to 70 percent of babies have oral bacteria surrounding them in the amniotic fluid,[19] though we aren't sure how much of that makes it into the baby. A baby gets their starter microbiome during delivery, and then grows and evolves their gut microbiome from the first feeding onward. Babies who pass through the vaginal canal get their mother's vaginal bacteria as a starter, whereas babies born by C-section tend to get bacteria from the hospital drapes and their mother's skin as their starter.[20] However, these differences do not seem to last past six months of age.

As babies drink breast milk or formula, their microbiome changes.[21] Complex oligosaccharides, found only in human breast milk, feed the bacteria that form the mucous lining of the intestines and make vitamin K. The oligosaccharides cannot be found in cow's milk or any formulas. The effect of breast milk versus formula is limited, however, because as babies reach the stage where they begin to eat solid foods and crawl, around six months old, their gut microbiome changes drastically. Each meal, each toy mouthed, each taste of dirt or sand provides a continuous series of new microbes and food for current microbes. After toddlerhood, the gut biome will largely stay the same unless antibiotics, a stomach illness, or an unbalanced diet throws it out of whack.

Dysbiosis of the Gut Biome

While there is no one correct microbiome, there are serious consequences when the gut microbiome has the wrong species, mix of species, or proportion of species. Imagine a painting class where the instructor tries to guide the students to create a beach landscape. Each painting completed in that class will be totally unique; one may be a quiet tropical beach with many palm trees and next to no waves, while another might feature a rocky ocean beach with a few surfers braving huge swells. However, if a student paints the ocean red or spills white paint all over their canvas, a passerby might not recognize either painting as a beach. The gut microbiome is like that. Each person's biome is unique, and lots of variations are workable and identifiable as healthy or normal. But a microbiome populated with the "wrong color" of strains or whited out by antibiotics will cause immune disease.

Remember that each microbe of the GI tract has specific dietary needs, and the only way for it to get its food is from whatever we eat. If we eat only fried food, some microbes will thrive while others will die. Throw off the delicate balance, and we will likely have a lot of the species of bacteria that recruit our immune receptors and cause inflammation.

Each microbe of the GI tract has specific dietary needs. If we eat only fried food, some microbes will thrive while others will die.

Our recent dietary shift to ever-increasing amounts of carbohydrates, particularly sugar, has also changed the balance of the oral microbiome[22] such that 60 to 90 percent of people experience tooth decay. The microbiome of a healthy mouth is populated by certain *Streptococcus* varieties that produce antibacterials and hydrogen peroxide that ensure their survival. But a carbohydrate-rich diet—combined with bad oral hygiene—facilitates the development of an acidic matrix on the teeth. *Streptococcus* cannot survive in this acidic environment, so new bacteria move in, generating even more acid and causing tooth decay.[23]

If dietary changes cause the mouth microbiome to become populated with a different type of bacterium called Gram-negative, the esophagus may become damaged. These bacteria thrive on carbs and sugar, creating lipopolysaccharides that bind to immune receptors and cause inflammation. These same bacteria also increase the nitrite levels in the esophagus, which react with excessive acid from the stomach (also caused by a low-fiber, high-sugar diet), possibly leading to esophageal cancer.[24]

Gut dysbiosis may also trigger localized allergic reactions, specifically in the esophagus. Eosinophilic esophagitis (EoE) is a chronic allergic inflammatory disease of the esophagus. While there is limited data, studies of children with EoE versus healthy children show shifts in their esophageal microbiomes. Scientists think that these bacteria promote the release of certain immune cells in the esophagus, which then trigger an allergic reaction, causing inflammation and injury.

Remember that allergic and autoimmune diseases like Crohn's, celiac disease, and IBD are all disproportionate reactions by the immune system to non-harmful antigens. Many studies have demonstrated that the gut microbiomes of infants and children with allergic and autoimmune diseases are quite distinct from those with healthy immune responses to food.[25] The bifidobacteria and lactobacilli in a healthy gut create short-chain fatty acids that increase your T regulatory cells, which keep the immune system calm. The intestinal microbes found in a dysbiotic gut will instead stimulate the immune system and train it to respond to non-harmful antigens, causing disease.

A relatively rare species called *Akkermansia* represents only 3 percent of the bacteria in the gut. This species plays an important role in communicating with cells in the gut lining and regulating mucus production. If we take this one species away, we can lose the ability to make mucus. Loss of *Akkermansia* can be a tipping point for a host of inflammation-related diseases and "leaky gut" conditions, in which the mucous lining fails to prevent antigens from seeping through the intestine.[26] Leaky gut has been implicated in a whole host of autoimmune and psychological disorders.

Finally, a breakdown or significant shift in the gut biome from what's most beneficial to a person may have profound effects on their physical and mental state. Studies in mice and rats have also shown that if an acid created by colon microbes is removed from their bodies, they develop immediate antisocial autism-like behaviors.[27] Luckily, changes that shift the gut microbes back into the direction of "normal" have proven effective in reducing or reversing certain behaviors related to autism.

Gut Dysbiosis and COVID-19

We've established with certainty that gut dysbiosis affects the immune system, and we recently saw this in action during the COVID-19 pandemic. Even in its earliest months—when the disease was still relatively misunderstood—doctors and scientists noticed how strange it was that some infected people recovered well while others got desperately sick and died. They began to notice a correlation between obesity and diabetes—both of which are linked to dysbiosis—but questioned why nondiabetic, slender, seemingly healthy people went down, too. Scientists looked for biomarkers that could help them predict who would get better on their own, knowing that if they could do so, they could create strategies to help prevent the most at risk from falling ill.

In early 2021—when the disease was everywhere and less mysterious than it had been initially—a study demonstrated that the composition of the intestinal and oral microbiome predicted with 92 percent and 84 percent accuracy, respectively, whether a patient would develop severe COVID-19 respiratory symptoms that would lead to death. If doctors combined symptoms, comorbidities, and the intestinal microbiota (particularly the presence of *Enterococcus faecalis* in stool), they could predict who would die with 96 percent accuracy.[28] In fact, the gut microbiome was the top predictor of COVID-19 disease severity—more than age or weight.

Even more interestingly, another study showed that gut microbiome composition was different in patients who caught COVID-19 compared with non-COVID-19.[29] Think of how babies who develop allergies have guts different from babies who don't. This is somewhat similar. This study reveals that the gut biome can tell you not only who gets severe COVID but who catches it at all!

Unfortunately, with this more recent disease, all we know right now is that the gut microbiomes of the COVID and non-COVID groups are different. We do not yet know which shifts made the critical difference. But you can believe that people are chasing this line of research to see if we can protect ourselves against the next pandemic!

....

We Need a New Way of Caring for Babies

I was recently talking to a fellow mom on the playground about the mission I've been on to learn more about our body's relationship to the microbiome. At some point between giving one son a snack and pushing another on the swings, I made a comment about how I'd recently read an article in *The New York Times* that stated that a full 95 percent of scientific research on the microbiome was published within the last decade.[30] We've known about our biomes for centuries, yet we've only just begun to look into them. Given how important the microbiome is to our immune systems, this seems shocking to me. My friend then said something that struck me.

"So over the last ten years," she remarked, "we've basically learned we have two immune systems, but we've been ignoring one of them."

I had never thought of it that way, but she was right. *The microbiome is like a second layer of the immune system.*

The microbiome and its effect on your baby's barriers are crucial to your child's health. It's imperative that we do everything to protect it. A healthy microbiome means a well child. Children who are constantly scratching and clawing at themselves aren't just a teensy bit itchy; they may have a case of eczema that—coupled with all the scratching—is causing their skin to become dysbiotic. I was shocked to discover the raw, itchy cracks in the folds of my son's arms were letting a bacterium as harmful as *S. aureus* seep into his body. When I discovered the connection between Leo's eczema and his food allergies, I was even more appalled that those cracks had then allowed his immune system to become overstimulated.

Recently, scientists have seen the connection between dysbiosis, barrier dysfunction, and immune disease play out in studies. The populations of Finland, Estonia, and Russian Karelia (the rural region of Russia bordering Finland) are genetically similar, but children in Finland have up to six times the rate of allergies and type 1 diabetes as Russian children. In Estonia, rates of childhood allergies and type 1 diabetes used to be similar to Karelia's, but as Estonia's economy and living standards grew following its independence from Russia in 1991, so, too, did its immune disease rates.

A longitudinal study[31] looking at the development of gut microbiomes in children from each of the three countries showed that Russian children's microbiomes in the first year were distinct from Finnish and Estonian children. Russian babies had significantly more *Bifidobacterium bifidum* and *Bifidobacterium longum,* the best breast milk metabolizers. Russian babies also had significantly higher rates of *E. coli* than of *Bacteroides dorei.* A lipid created by *B. dorei* is far more likely to generate an immune response than the same lipid created by *E. coli,* which is more likely to drive immune tolerance.

After age one, the gut microbiomes of babies from all three countries started to look the same, but clearly the damage had already been done in this critical development time frame. For the first year of life, Russian babies had "better" gut bacteria that prevented the onset of allergies and type 1 diabetes.

The gut difference was despite the fact that Finnish mothers were more likely to breastfeed and breastfed on average two months longer. Scientists concluded that the useful *E. coli, B. bifidum,* and *B. longum* were missing from Finnish children because of either antibiotics, Finnish hygiene practices, diet, or environment. (Interestingly, the day care facilities in Finland started building their own "forests," and it drastically improved kids' immune systems.)

Reading research like this made clear that dysbiosis of the microbiome was probably at the root of Leo's years of suffering, too. As I spoke to scientists and scoured the internet and scientific journals, it suddenly became clear to me that something the rural families in Russian Karelia did fostered a diverse infant microbiome, while the practices of the economically advanced Finnish and Estonian families hurt it. Was the "modern" advice parents like me had followed since we'd first discovered we were expecting actually hurting our children? While trying to foster a healthy, happy child, was I doing things that were incredibly damaging to my baby's microbiome?

The answer is yes.

Today, I can search "infant bathing practices" or "how to treat a childhood fever" in leading research journals and invariably find new studies suggesting that much of what I had done with Leo was all wrong. Humans have evolved over thousands of years with certain microbes, and these microbes are a key part of the magic that allows humans to thrive. Allergic and autoimmune diseases develop when we stop doing our part in the deal to keep them healthy. I had let Leo's microbiome become dysbiotic and thus had helped damage his precious barrier.

The research that has been released since Leo was born shows that you shouldn't bathe a baby for two weeks after birth because it strips their skin of healthy bacteria—but we bathed Leo the first day. Another paper says to actively treat cradle cap with antifungal shampoo and to immediately care for even mild eczema with topical steroids or trigger removal, but we had let both progress to the point of letting an infection settle in and needing antibiotics. As soon as Leo showed eczema, we should have fed him every allergenic food to train his body to tolerate them, not avoided such foods. And during his immune development window, we should have been aggressive about recognizing his gut dysbiosis and healing it instead of hoping it would resolve on its own.

When I compared the recommendations from these papers to my notes from doctor's visits and even pictures saved on my phone, all I could see was a list of mistakes. No single decision was enough to cause Leo's trifecta of eczema, asthma, and food allergies, but possibly the sum of them tipped his immune system into a lifelong imbalance that would mean he could never eat a birthday cake or kiss someone without fear.

In the following chapters, we'll discuss each of the major players in barrier dysfunction and dysbiosis: antibiotics, baby care, diet, and environment. We'll also cover what the current research tells us about how to find a pathway back to health. While our understanding of barrier dysfunction and the microbiome's effect on our health is still coming into focus, the overall picture is quite clear: our goal as parents must be to promote and support our children's barriers and get them back into shape if they are damaged. We have to take care of our babies' microbes, and that means setting them up with a healthy microbiome at birth and maintaining it throughout—especially during the first three years.

CHAPTER THREE
································

Antibiotics Change Everything

Common Misconception:
If your child has an ear infection,
you need an antibiotic to cure it.
···

About 90 percent of children get ear infections, most often between the ages of six months and four years. There is no rapid test to determine what pathogen is causing an ear infection, so many doctors will prescribe an antibiotic immediately, thinking it's better to be safe than sorry. Unfortunately, most of the time antibiotics are completely ineffective for ear infections because roughly 80 percent of ear infections are not caused by bacteria but instead by a virus. When your child develops an ear infection, hold off on the antibiotics until necessary and treat their pain with Tylenol or Advil instead.

The average child receives ten courses of antibiotics before getting to kindergarten.[1] My son didn't have it quite as bad, but by eighteen months he had been prescribed antibiotics at least four times. The first time was for a respiratory infection, the second for a high fever, the third to clear up a skin infection, and a fourth for an ear infection not long after he started day care. Each time, it felt like the right thing to do. As a worried parent, I wanted my baby to get better.

What my husband and I didn't know was that using antibiotics when it's not *absolutely necessary* can actually make a child sick longer, can cause significant complications like diarrhea or stomach upset, may increase the chances you'll have to visit the doctor a second time, and will most certainly affect their microbiome.

Using antibiotics when it's not *absolutely necessary* can actually make a child sick longer and can cause significant complications like diarrhea or stomach upset.

The word *antibiotic* literally means "against life." Antibiotics are critical life-saving, bacteria-killing nuclear weapons that have a dizzying ability to wage war against an infection. But they are also indiscriminate. Like the bomb, they kill everything in their path, including bacteria beneficial to you. They can make it to any part of your body—from your gut to your brain to your reproductive organs—and most parents should find this terrifying. The problem is that even the most educated, well-meaning moms and dads haven't been given this knowledge. I sure wasn't. When Leo came home from preschool tugging at his ears and crying in pain, I didn't think twice about giving him spoonfuls of amoxicillin twice a day for ten days. I just didn't want to see my son suffer.

We are only beginning to grapple with the damage antibiotics have caused in our children. Worse, we are only now realizing these drugs' sheer scope. Antibiotics are *everywhere,* even in places many people don't realize. Our food—specifically meat and dairy—drip antibiotics into us every day. The chemicals on the antibacterial wipes we used on every surface in the house during the COVID-19 pandemic made their way into our children's bloodstreams, as did those in the hand sanitizer ubiquitous in every classroom and store. The Neosporin antibiotic ointment we rub on tiny boo-boos kills infection-causing bacteria, but it also destroys the beneficial organisms that may help your child heal. And when our kids get sick, we give them more courses of antibiotics than they truly need, causing dysbiosis and far worse conditions than the infection we want to cure.

We need to rid our homes and plates of microbiome killers and be far more careful with how we medicate our children. The overuse of antibiotics has become a crisis, and the time to deal with it is now.

....

The Discovery That Changed Life Expectancy

Before antibiotics, one in ten women died in childbirth, many of them from infections that began days after their children were born, when they assumed they were safe from any danger. Tetanus, pneumonia, and urinary tract, sinus, and eye infections could all be deadly for children, and over 90 percent of children with bacterial meningitis died. The few who survived had severe and lasting disabilities. Strep throat—which is a complete nonissue today because it isn't contagious after one day of antibiotics—was often fatal, and ear infections frequently spread to the brain.

All that changed with antibiotics.

It is easy to forget that less than 150 years ago, the idea that tiny single-celled organisms could make us sick—much less keep us healthy—sounded absurd. Around the dawn of the twentieth century, though, German physician and bacteriologist Robert Koch demonstrated that you could take a bacterium from someone sick, grow it on a dish, then give it to a healthy person and make *them* sick in the same way. With this discovery, people finally began to accept the "germ theory" of disease, and scientists threw their energy at finding ways to rid us of bacteria, the supposed source of all illness. Popular efforts started with water purification and personal hygiene, but soon the scientific establishment zeroed in on cures for infections.

Then the world changed in 1928 following an accident in Scottish researcher Alexander Fleming's lab.[2] After returning from a two-week vacation, Fleming was disappointed to see that a spot of mold had contaminated one of the culture plates he was using to grow staphylococcus. When he looked closer, he could see that the small fuzz of fungus on the plate was surrounded by empty space with no bacterial growth. Clearly, the mold held real significance. If it could kill bacteria on a culture plate, could it do the same in living organisms?

It could. This specific mold, eventually identified as *Penicillium notatum,* secretes a chemical compound that Fleming named penicillin. Penicillin disrupts proteins in bacterial cell walls, killing them as they try to divide. By the end of World War II, the discovery of penicillin and years of international efforts to figure out how to produce it at scale meant that significantly fewer soldiers died of battle wounds than did in World War I.

The amazing success of penicillin at bringing people back from illnesses and injuries that used to mean certain death allowed Alexander Fleming to win the Nobel Prize in Physiology or Medicine in 1945. Eventually scientists grew penicillin from other microorganisms, leading to the general category of antibiotics. In the decades that followed, scientists created strep-tomycin (used to treat tuberculosis), chloramphenicol (for conjunctivitis, meningitis, bubonic plague, and typhus), eryth-romycin (for everything from chest infections to sexually trans-mitted diseases), vancomycin (for staph and intestinal infections), and many others.

....

Antibiotics Are Everywhere

Today, everybody understands the power antibiotics hold to treat infections. One December, my sister and brother-in-law were coming to visit with their twin toddlers. Scott and I were about to have eight people staying in our house, including four kids under two years old. A few days before my sister's family arrived, though, I developed a sinus headache and a fever. I ignored it for a day or so until I woke up one morning thinking, *There's no way I can see anyone.* I visited the doctor that afternoon, and she gave me an antibiotic prescription. Within a day of starting it, I felt almost back to normal. The effects were strong and immediate, and I was cured seemingly without any side effects.

It's no wonder that doctors seeing similarly magic results in patients with otherwise life-threatening infections would start prescribing antibiotics more and more, even when they lacked a confirmed diagnosis of bacterial infection and even when the use of antibiotics did not necessarily produce a better outcome than other treatments. It seemed like a logical choice to be "bet-ter safe than sorry."

Unfortunately, today we are learning that the effects of anti-biotic overuse can instead be "sorry rather than safe."

A recent study in *JAMA: The Journal of the American Medical Association* showed that despite clear evidence that antibiotics should never be prescribed for acute bronchitis—a wheezing, deep cough that is always viral—about 70 percent of bronchitis patients from 1996 to 2010 received antibiotic prescriptions.[3] These statistics are much worse in children, who often get respiratory infections and ear infections, the two most common problems treated by primary care physicians.

Yet nearly 80 percent of these infections are caused by viruses, which means that antibacterials will have no effect. In addition, most bacterial infections will clear on their own, without treatment.

It's easy to say that physicians overprescribe antibiotics and that they should have no problem limiting their use. But while telling if someone is sick is fairly straightforward, it's not as simple to determine who will clear out the infection on their own and which baby's ear infection is viral versus bacterial. The fluid that pools around the eardrum in an ear infection can be cultured, but that procedure requires local or general anesthesia. You can't just do it right there in the pediatrician's office between your child's vision test and the lollipop they pick up at checkout. Instead, in the interest of money, patient care, and time, doctors often prefer to prescribe an antibiotic and hope it works. It's also not possible to know which baby will develop complications from fighting off an infection, called rheumatic fever, and end up incredibly sick weeks later. Again, better safe than sorry, so amoxicillin it is.

Yet, we have to try to do better.

Every time infants and children are given "just in case" antibiotics for respiratory infections, it starts to add up. Toddlers in general will have received three prescriptions for antibiotics during their first eighteen months. After that age, an individual is likely to be prescribed a little fewer than one course of antibiotics *per year* until they are well into adulthood. That's almost thirty courses of antibiotics by age forty.[4] Every single time you take an antibiotic, it indiscriminately wipes out a huge percentage of the bacteria throughout your body. Remember how the microbiome makes up 99 percent of our genes? Well, taking a course of antibiotics could be like ripping out half of your genome. How well did things go the last time you had only half of an instruction manual?

What happens after you finish up your antibiotics? Option one is that your microbiome goes back to the way it was before. The volume of bacterial species in your gut, on your skin, and elsewhere will have greatly decreased, but as you heal, they will repopulate in the same manner they did before. Think of this as a forest fire in an old-growth pine forest. The fire may destroy all the trees, but tiny pinecones buried under the soot will grow into tall pines someday. Option two is that all the same species come back but in a different balance. After a different forest fire, all the same trees may grow back, but trees that grow faster can overtake more area than they had before the fire. Option three is that the mix fundamentally changes. If a destructive fire takes out a rare species, that species could simply disappear forever.

Every single time you take an antibiotic, it indiscriminately wipes out a huge percentage of the bacteria throughout your body.

Option three is the cautionary tale of a microbe like *Bacteroides fragilis*. Although it makes up less than 1 percent of the microbes in the colon, it produces a polysaccharide that regulates immune macrophage cells, preventing them from overreacting. If every bacterial species' population in the colon is cut in half, *B. fragilis* could get so reduced that it is simply lost. Studies of ulcerative colitis in animals have shown that this extinction creates immune system deficiencies that can lead to widespread damaging intestinal inflammation.[5]

Taking unnecessary courses of antibiotics is bad, but it almost pales as a source of worry compared to the antibiotics used in our food. An estimated 80 percent of all antibiotics by weight in the United States are used in agriculture and fed to live-stock.[6] There are two reasons large industrial farms rely on these drugs. The first is that they hold animals in buildings and pens with far too many other animals. When animals live in such tight quarters that they can't even turn around, much less move in one direction or another, they soil themselves repeatedly. And because of how densely packed these cages and pens are, there's no efficient way to eliminate the waste from the housing area. Healthy bacteria in the stomach can become massively infectious bacteria in animal waste, so to avoid losing a herd to disease, industrial farms add antibiotics to their livestock feed.

The second reason industrial farms use antibiotics is that it tends to fatten the animals faster, creating more meat and more profit for the farm. It is believed that the use of antibiotics in animals and humans kills the colon bacteria that metabolize food into vitamins and minerals, making eating an inefficient process. Without proper calorie extraction, animals consume larger quantities of food to get the same amount of nutrients. They then store more food as fat. What does a bigger, fatter animal mean? More meat and more profit.

Some of the antibiotics livestock take in end up in the water supply as the animals clear them out of their system. But those that don't simply flush through the animal end up as residue in the food we get. Take milk, for example. Milk can legally have up to 100 micrograms of tetracycline per kilogram, and a 1990 report showed that 30 to 80 percent of milk samples had detectable levels of antibiotics.[7] In addition, a not insignificant amount of the food at the grocery store will exceed the allowable limits because testing and enforcement cannot keep up with the demands. Since the passage of the 2011 Food Safety Modernization Act, the FDA has received less than half of the money it needs to ensure the safety of the food supply.

The overuse of antibiotics isn't limited to livestock. For around fifty years, farmers have used antibiotics to control bacterial disease in crops such as apples and pears.[8] However, an investigation[9] by the Food and Agricultural Organization of the United Nations (FAO), the World Organisation for Animal Health (OIE), and the World Health Organization (WHO) revealed that, out of 158 countries questioned about their monitoring of antibiotic use in agriculture, only 3 percent actively tracked and assessed their use. In some countries in South Asia, for example, an estimated 63 tons of streptomycin and 7 tons of tetracycline are sprayed on rice crops annually. In a few regions, 10 percent of rice crops contained antibiotics. Antibiotics are also being used to rid crops of pests—despite the fact that these drugs have no effect against anything but bacteria.

Our kids' microbiomes are foundational to their ability to discern microscopic friend from foe, yet we assail those microbiomes annually with antibiotic medications and daily with milk, fruits, grains, and meat riddled with antibiotics. Still wondering why allergic and autoimmune diseases are on the rise?

....

Making Better Antibiotics

One solution to the widespread damage from antibiotics is to find ways to target the exact bacterial species that is causing an infection. *Streptococcus pyogenes* is a species that usually lives happily and harmlessly inside the noses of up to 20 percent of people. Yet it can also be virulent, causing strep throat, scarlet fever, "flesh-eating disease," and rheumatic fever. Wouldn't it be nice if we could target *S. pyogenes* and eradicate it entirely? Unfortunately, antibiotics are nuclear bombs, not snipers, so selective killing isn't possible.

Even if selective killing were possible, though, it wouldn't necessarily be the best route to take. Most bacterial species aren't "enemies" like *S. pyogenes*; they may be helpful one day and deadly the next. Take *Staphylococcus epidermidis*, for example. It's the beneficial bacterium on our skin that talks to our immune system and prevents *Staphylococcus aureus* from pouring biotoxin through our cells. However, it is also the leading cause of sepsis, or blood infection, in the hospital. *S. epidermidis* is commonly picked up by catheters and other medical devices inserted through the skin, where it grows colonies and sends little clusters floating off through the bloodstream.

S. epidermidis infections damage tissues and lead to organ failure, and they can quickly become deadly. The mortality rate of sepsis hovers around 40 percent, and it's estimated that one in five neonatal deaths around the world can be attributed to it.[10] Sepsis is also extremely difficult to treat because *S. epidermidis* creates a biofilm protective coating that allows it to cling to surfaces and avoid antibiotics. While this is a trick that lets it beat out competition on the skin, fighting it also requires huge doses of these drugs to stop it.

The problem is that destroying it in the bloodstream almost definitely also destroys it on the skin, disturbing the delicate balance of microbes that protect you. Even targeting (sniping) and killing a specific bacterium like *S. epidermidis* would mean unpleasant side effects. Some people might develop temporary rosacea, whereas others might experience adult-onset eczema, allergies, or worse.

....

Antibiotics and Your Baby

About 90 percent of children get ear infections[11] (otitis media), most often between ages six months and four years. Children with acute ear infections have fever and ear pain, and if they're too young to speak, they may pull on their ears to signal their discomfort. The effusion that may accompany an illness is caused by extra fluid in the middle ear, and it can cause difficulty hearing or headaches. Children often get ear infections with effusion after having a cold or viral infection.

Ear infections are the most common childhood infection for which antibiotics are prescribed. Yet roughly 80 percent of them do not require antibiotics because they are caused by viruses or because the infection will clear on its own.[12] Worse, 4 to 10 percent of children who receive these antibiotics have subsequent problems, including vomiting, diarrhea, and rashes.[13]

Ear infections are far from the only illness for which antibiotics are prescribed. Other common infections that don't benefit from antibiotic treatment include colds, the flu, bronchitis, most coughs, some sinus infections, and stomach flus. Yet almost all parents have a story about their children or their friend's child receiving a course of antibiotics for one of these conditions. I'm one of them. When he was one, my son woke up with a fever. I took him to the doctor, who couldn't find a discernible cause. The pediatrician prescribed an antibiotic and the fever cleared up, but I still wonder if children's acetaminophen wouldn't have had the same effect.

How do you prevent unnecessary use of antibiotics in your baby? The first part of the answer is to reduce the risk that your child gets sick in the first place.

1. **Wash your child's hands with soap and water, not hand sanitizer.**

   Before you or your baby eats, wash your hands. It is not for nothing that washing hands is considered the single most effective way to prevent infections. Handwashing with soap for at least twenty seconds removes germs, and don't forget to wash the front and the back of your hands. Also scrub between your fingers and under your nails, where pathogens can hide.

   A friend's daughter frequently came down with pinworms, which are small clear parasites that live harmlessly in everyone's intestines and colons. When a child wipes after going to the bathroom, however, their fingernails may scrape up the eggs that pinworms lay near the anus. When children eat (often with their dirty little fingers), they ingest those eggs, and the pinworms multiply more than they should. At night, the new batch of pinworms exits the anus and lays *more* eggs, which causes your child to have significant itching.

   Pinworm infections are easy to treat with an over-the-counter antiparasitic, but my friend's daughter experienced this one too many times during kindergarten. My friend started cutting her daughter's fingernails weekly, never letting them grow long, and monitored her child's handwashing every time she went to the bathroom. Her daughter never experienced another itchy pinworm infection.

   If handwashing can rid you of pinworms, just think what else it can do!

   Even though you want to protect your kid's microbiome, you should still wash their hands, because soap and water will not destroy large swaths of bacteria. Soap works by surrounding dirt and oil and dislodging it from the skin. As you rub and rinse your hands, the dirt and germs will be washed away along with the soap.

I know it can be hard to wash a child's hands before eating when you are not inside. If possible, pack homemade soap-and-water-infused towels in plastic bags and keep them in your backpack, your purse, the car, or your child's backpack or lunch box. Otherwise, feed your child with a spoon to limit their consumption of unhelpful pathogens that

> You should still wash your kids' hands because soap and water will not destroy their microbiome. Soap works by surrounding dirt and oil and dislodging it from the skin.

live on their fingers and nails. Try to be aware of what these germs might be, too. The microbes that your kid picks up when playing on a swing set or attending day care are probably more pathogenic than helpful. The bacteria from dirt in your no-pesticide garden, however, are probably fine.

Do not use hand sanitizer or baby wipes on a child's hands if you can avoid it. Hand sanitizers other than those with ethyl alcohol are not considered safe by the FDA. Hand sanitizer with ethyl alcohol must also be used properly, which means you need to let it air-dry in order to dehydrate the germs. If you choose to use sanitizer or wipes, just know that you will be left with the chemicals from the hand sanitizer or baby wipe on your hands, which may destroy the commensal bacteria on your skin and can enter the body as you eat and damage internal bacteria.

2. Breastfeed if possible, at least for two months. Then vaccinate and get flu shots.

Before the pneumococcal vaccine was given to all babies, the most common cause of ear and respiratory infections was the bacterium *Streptococcus pneumoniae*. Before a baby is old enough to be vaccinated, breast milk contains immune cells and provides immune protection to a baby.[14] After babies receive their first set of vaccinations for bacterial diseases (pneumococcal conjugate for *S. pneumoniae*; Hib for *Haemophilus influenzae* type b; Tdap for tetanus, diphtheria, and pertussis), a large number of bacterial infections that would require antibiotics can be avoided. We will talk more about breastfeeding in chapter 4.

Getting the flu shot every year will reduce the risk of the flu. Children as young as six months old can receive the shot, and there is even a nasal spray vaccine that can be given to children starting when they are two. The flu is a common cause of pneumonia (a bacterial lung infection that sets in when the body is beaten down by a virus), especially among younger children, so reducing the risk of a viral infection reduces the chances of inappropriate antibiotics.

3. **Avoid bottle feeding your baby when they are lying down.** It is very tempting to feed babies a bottle while they are lying on their back. I developed horrible neck pain from holding my babies up to the breast to nurse, so I completely understand the temptation. Many women also slouch over or tilt to one side when they breastfeed, and this can cause back pain. Placing a baby on a pillow can help, as can bottle feeding when a baby is put in the correct position.

   This correct position is *not* flat on their back. When babies drink from a bottle while they're lying down, the milk can pool in the mouth and flow back into the middle ear, where it can cause infection. Try placing your baby in a reclined seat, sitting them up with pillows, or, if they're stable enough not to tip over, let them sit in their high chair or on the floor.

4. **Do not smoke; secondhand smoke can increase the risk of ear infections.**[15]

   Having a family member who smokes raises the risk of ear infections for children in the same house. Smoking causes chronic inflammation that triggers the immune system, and it damages tissues in the nose and throat—not only of the smoker but also of anyone inhaling secondhand smoke. A triggered immune system is more prone to ear infections, and children—whose inner ears have a different shape that doesn't drain well—are at higher risk for them. Do not smoke near children or let them get near anyone who is smoking.

5. **Pay attention to a possible cow's milk allergy.**

   An undiagnosed cow's milk allergy is often associated with an infant's developing recurring ear infections with effusion.[16] (*Effusion* in this case means fluid in the middle ear. It does not necessarily mean fluid coming out of the ear.) Children with food allergies and asthma are thought to be more likely to get ear infections as a result of ingesting the allergen. However, it's worth pointing out that repeated antibiotic use from previous ear infections also increases the risk of allergy. It's not clear which comes first. If a baby younger than six months drinks formula rather than breast milk exclusively, they take in the formula's number one ingredient: cow's milk. Many children with a milk allergy will present symptoms other than ear infections, including eczema, lung, and stomach issues, but if an infant or child has recurring ear infections, the possibility of food allergies should be

   > If an infant or child has recurring ear infections, the possibility of food allergies should be explored. Elimination of the allergenic foods might prevent another course of antibiotics.

explored. Elimination of the allergenic foods might prevent another course of antibiotics.

....

Treating Infections

If we are to reduce the unnecessary use of antibiotics, we have to be judicious, careful, and informed, treating each prescription for antibiotics like the powerful and dangerous (when misused) tool that it is.

The current American Academy of Pediatrics (AAP) guidelines[17] say that before diagnosing an ear infection, a doctor must see:

1. Moderate bulging of the tympanic membrane (eardrum) or ear drainage not linked to known inflammation

   Or

2. Mild bulging AND intense redness of the tympanic membrane, plus (in the case of a baby) holding, tugging, or rubbing of the ear.

The AAP's guidelines suggest that antibiotics should be given only if an ear infection is definitively diagnosed, meaning they meet the criteria above. If one is definitely present, the patient should be categorized based on illness severity (severe earache, earache lasting more than 48 hours, or temperature higher than 103°F), spread of infection (both ears versus one ear), and age (less than two months versus two years or older). Children with more severe symptoms, both ears involved, and under age two are more likely to benefit from antibiotics. If your baby does not meet the criteria for needing antibiotics, do not use them.

With children under two or those with severe infections, doctors may want to use antibiotics to protect a child's hearing or avoid larger issues like an infection of the mastoid bone, which is located behind the ear. On the other hand, if antibiotics are used when they're not truly needed, they can cause abdominal pain, diarrhea, rashes, and in the worst cases, *Clostridioides difficile* (*C. diff*) colitis.

If your child has an ear infection that may benefit from antibiotics, have a discussion with your doctor about the pros and cons. At least half of bacterial ear infections heal on their own, so sometimes a wait-and-see approach is the best course to take. If your course of action is one of "watchful waiting," you should allow your child's immune system two to three days to fight the infection and give them plenty of rest, extra fluids, and mild pain relievers to ease their symptoms. It can be extremely hard to watch your child in pain for two days before their fever breaks or they start to feel better, but it is significantly better than hurting their microbiome unnecessarily. Another trick that may make parents feel better is to get a prescription from the doctor but wait to fill it. For a lot of us, knowing that we can get the amoxicillin quickly if things haven't gotten better in three days brings just enough peace to wait it out.

I asked the team of doctors at Society Hill Pediatrics in Philadelphia how they handle the ambiguous cases. One pediatrician responded, "I would likely treat a child less than twenty-four months with antibiotics if I diagnose an ear infection. For children eighteen to twenty-four months, I engage the parents in a discussion about waiting a few days if the child has no other signs or symptoms, such as fever or obvious pain. I would also be more inclined to treat a child of any age with antibiotics if he or she has a history of frequent ear infections or has had any complication from an ear infection, or if there is history of requiring pressure-equalizing tubes for chronic ear infections."

If you truly feel something isn't right with your child, though, don't feel you have to keep waiting. When Leo broke out into hives from eating eggs before his first birthday, I was so worried about appearing like a Nervous Nellie to our pediatrician that I didn't call her as soon as my gut told me to.

In short, don't jump to conclusions, but trust your parental instincts. As with anything in parenting, balance is key.

> If you truly feel something isn't right with your child, don't feel you have to keep waiting to call your doctor.

While ear infections are the biggest cause of antibiotic prescriptions written for children, watchful waiting is important when it comes to other illnesses, too. For sinus infections, antibiotics should be avoided unless a child has a fever of 102 for more than three days, green nasal discharge, distinct facial pain, a cough that isn't gone after ten days, or symptoms that steadily worsen instead of plateauing. Sore throats (pharyngitis) are almost never bacterial, and a rapid test (a quick swab in the back of a child's throat) for streptococcus bacteria can be used to tell if the sore throat is viral or is actually strep. Viral sore throats are typically associated with a phlegmy cough and a lot of snot, but you should ask your pediatrician for a test if you want to know for sure. Antibiotics should never be used for viral sore throats. Finally, common colds, coughs, and acute bronchitis should never be prescribed antibiotics, as they are not caused by bacteria.

I am friends with a pediatric ER doctor named Marleny Franco, MD, who works at the Children's Hospital of Philadelphia. I was speaking to her recently about my concern that antibiotics are overprescribed, and she told me: "In ten years of practicing ER medicine, only a handful of parents have questioned me for prescribing antibiotics. I remember them because they stuck out. On the other hand, I get questioned all the time for *not* writing an antibiotic prescription that isn't needed."

In order to care for your baby's microbiome, *be the parent who questions antibiotics.*

Dr. Franco added that she understands that many parents bring their kids in because of "fever phobia,"[18] and that seeing their child red-faced, hot, and in obvious distress can make any mother or father desperate for something to help. Just know that a temperature below 100.3 is technically not a fever, and that while fever is a sign of an infection, the number itself is not an indicator of severity. Parents hate the idea of allowing their child to have a fever—possibly for several days—but a fever is a normal, healthy sign that the immune system is working, and we have to let the immune system do its job. If we all practiced more judicious antibiotic use, we and our children may feel pain in the short term, but we will see huge payoffs in the long run.

Another pediatrician, Katie Lockwood, said, "As parents, we want to offer our children something, anything, to make their pain or discomfort go away as fast as possible. Giving our children medicine makes us feel empowered in that we are doing something, but we need to make sure we aren't doing unintentional harm. Judicious use of antibiotics is important so that we can avoid unnecessary risk and trust that antibiotics will work when they are needed most."

> **For sinus infections, antibiotics should be avoided unless a child has a fever of 102 for more than three days, green nasal discharge, distinct facial pain, a cough that isn't gone after ten days, or symptoms that steadily worsen instead of plateauing.**

....

Stopping Antibiotics When
They Are Not Needed

The most persistent myth about antibiotics is that you always have to finish a given course. If the instructions on the bottle read, "Use for ten days," most people believe they cannot stop after three days if they are feeling better. They think that ending the course will allow the infection to come raging back, possibly even stronger than it was before.

This misconception comes from a lack of understanding of how antibiotics work. The goal of antibiotics is to reduce overall bacterial levels to the point that *your immune system* can kill the infection. Antibiotics should not work by themselves to remove an infection. *You*, or *your baby*, are the leader of your battle against illness. Once your baby is feeling better and their symptoms are gone, this means that their immune system is done fighting the infection. This is not just me talking, either. Scientists and doctors now agree that it is safe—indeed, from the perspective of microbiome destruction, safer—to stop antibiotics as soon as they are not needed.[19]

> The goal of antibiotics is to reduce overall bacterial levels to the point that *your immune system* can kill the infection.

I want to be clear that when I say you should avoid finishing a course of antibiotics, I am talking about antibiotics alone, *not* other prescriptions your child might need. In the months after Leo had the asthma attack that sent him to the hospital and left me wondering if child services would knock on my door, my son experienced at least three more asthma attacks that took multiple doses of inhaled steroids as well as oral steroids to treat. Each episode drained us further, yet I continued to oppose the idea of daily steroids. I couldn't stand the thought of my child on a daily medication for the rest of his life. What I didn't understand was that each course of rescue steroids for a flare was the equivalent in medication dosage of *five years* of preventative daily medication. By resisting daily medication so stubbornly, I had allowed my child to receive twenty-five years' worth of it.

In short, be careful with antibiotics, and follow your doctor's advice with any other prescriptions your child receives.

....

The Problem of Antibiotic Resistance

Each year in the United States, 2.8 million people become infected with antibiotic-resistant bacteria, and 35,000 of them die as a result.[20] The main reason these microbes become tolerant of the antibiotics used to treat them is because of antibiotic overuse. The more we use antibiotics, the more bacteria are killed—but some always survive. These super-strong bacteria then multiply, and in a perverse version of survival of the fittest, become more widespread, minimizing the effectiveness of antibiotics with every subsequent dose.

Antibiotic use was rising steadily in Sweden during the 1980s and 1990s, causing an increase in antibiotic-resistant bacteria. A group of doctors within Sweden's national health system decided they had to reverse this trend. The Swedish Strategic Programme Against Antibiotic Resistance (Strama)[21] was founded in 1995 to create national and local strategies to reduce antibiotic use. Between 1992 and 2016, antibiotics prescriptions decreased by 43 percent overall, and for children under four, antibiotics prescriptions fell by 73 percent. Sweden now has one of the lowest levels of prescriptions per person or animal and the fewest issues with antibiotic resistance.

A World Health Organization review noted a few important steps that Sweden took in preparation for this sweeping change. All doctors, hospitals, and farms were required to report every use of antibiotics, and this data was collected, analyzed, and reported at a local and national level. Sweden made a concerted effort to educate the media and general public (in multiple languages!) on why people should try to avoid antibiotics. They also continued to track outcomes of cases where antibiotics were not prescribed to ensure that infection rates and bad outcomes were not increasing.

All the way back in 1986, Sweden banned the use of antimicrobial growth promoters in livestock and fisheries. Even with that ban, Sweden has reported no increase in infections in slaughtered pigs, beef, turkeys, and broiler chickens. This reduction in antibiotic use on farms did require a lot of hard work, and for a period of time, there were significant issues with piglet production. However, improved management techniques meant that by 1999, only 5 percent of piglet-producing herds used antibiotic-medicated feed. Sweden proved that antibiotics in feed are not necessary if livestock are managed properly.

For the sake of protecting people from antibiotic-resistant bacteria as well as from a whole host of dysbiosis-related diseases, we can and should reduce our use of antibiotics. Sweden proved it can be done. Unfortunately, without national policy in the United States, parents like you and me *must* take personal responsibility to avoid antibiotics when they are not needed and "vote with our dollars" to buy antibiotic-free meats, dairy, and fish whenever possible. We must stop courses of antibiotics when we or our children are clearly doing better, and we should avoid topical antibacterials like Neosporin, hand sanitizers, and antibacterial soap. Because they are *everywhere,* I'll talk about antibiotic cleansers and cleaning products more in chapter 6.

Let's be very clear that antibiotics should be used when they are necessary. Bacteria can cause harmful infections, and antibiotics absolutely save lives. It's only their unnecessary use that we need to avoid, and as the Swedish example shows, their use is unnecessary in probably three out of four cases.

Your baby's microbiome is developing and changing rapidly during the first three years and laying the foundation for your child's subsequent immune system and lifelong health. Preventing destructive fires of the microbiome is important, but it is equally crucial to make decisions that help create a strong forest in the first place.

CHAPTER FOUR

....

Baby Care the First
Six Months

Common Misconception:
Infant vaccines cause allergic disease.

....

The fundamental reason infant vaccines cannot cause allergic disease is that vaccines activate different cells than the immune cells that overreact in allergic diseases. Each immune team—Team 1, Team 2, or Team 17—responds to viruses, parasites, or bacteria, respectively. A bacterial vaccine will teach Team 17 to respond to that bacterium, but bacterial vaccines will not cause Team 1 or Team 2 cells to do anything because it's not their job. Many people blame vaccines for allergic diseases because vaccination requires injecting a kind of pathogen into the bloodstream, thus causing an immune response. But again, the pathogen that is injected is a thing we *want* the body to react to.

One of the stranger things about becoming a parent is how much emphasis is put on pregnancy and childbirth as opposed to actually raising your baby. I took a multi-week, fourteen-hour class about labor and delivery, but I was only *in* labor for eleven hours. Compare that to the class I took on infant care, which covered bathing, swaddling, feeding, and postpartum recovery. It lasted about one hour.

The fact is that the United States is one of the few developed nations in the world that doesn't provide interventions for new parents outside of pediatrician visits. New parents in Finland receive at least 164 days of paid parental leave and a box of sixty baby care essentials, including blankets, bibs, and snowsuits. My boys got a hat and a few samples of formula, and I got six paid weeks (42 days) off. I spent much of those weeks "off" still working. My sister in London was visited regularly by a nurse who wasn't shy about inspecting her house for dangers and asking questions to make sure she and my brother-in-law knew what they were doing. The National Health Service does this for all new parents, free of cost. In the United States, we have no guaranteed parental leave and no subsidized childcare. Instead, we have expensive day care centers, baby books that offer general advice, and pediatricians who are deeply caring but often overworked.

Our system lets too many avoidable things through the cracks, too. For example, every baby spits up occasionally, but before he was six months old Leo regurgitated a surprising amount after every single meal. I was concerned, so I went to my computer to find out if I should take him to the doctor. My internet search of "baby spit-up—how much is normal" told me to measure the amount Leo regurgitated and that a few tablespoons or more should raise a red flag. After the next meal, I scooped up his spit-up, measured it, and realized it was definitely less than Google said I should worry about. Just to be sure, I researched spit-up in a few of the baby books I had on my shelf. They all suggested excessive spit-up wasn't a problem unless Leo arched his back in pain and cried after meals. He never did that.

Yet I knew deep down that the spit-up *was* a problem. We always had muslin squares, burp cloths, bibs, towels, and extra clothes at the ready, and I felt like I did laundry twice as much as most new moms. I also have a particular memory of my best friend's mother coming to visit and catching Leo's spit-up with a dishrag. As she handed him back to me, I could see the worry in her eyes.

"You know," she said kindly, "if you're nursing and eating cruciferous vegetables like cauliflower and brussels sprouts, they can cause gas and bloating. That makes your baby spit up. Have you tried eliminating them from your diet?"

I cut out brussels sprouts and cauliflower, and it didn't help.

Looking back, I realize that my friend's mom's well-meaning advice, coupled with all those dishrags and towels, should have been a clear sign that something was wrong with Leo. But no book, article, or doctor mentioned that he might be having a kind of allergic reaction—or what that condition indicated about his immune system.

In fact, science has now fully established that I should have seen the spit-up for what it was: a clear sign of gastrointestinal epithelial dysfunction. His gut barrier was broken, and no quantity of burp cloths could fix that. If I had known what his problem was, I could have treated it by nurturing and healing his microbiome. The younger a baby is, the better the odds of reversing damage or preventing future damage, and because Leo was only a few months old, his immune system was still very much a work in progress.

The habits parents put in place and the choices they make

during their child's first six months can either foster strong barriers and a healthy immune system or set off a chain reaction of allergic responses that takes years to control. I accidentally let my own child rack up allergic diseases, but there's no reason you have to do the same. Revisiting basic baby care and understanding how it helps or harms your child's barriers and microbiome is not as hard as you think. In this chapter, I'll walk you through some of the most basic early childcare activities—including breastfeeding, vaccinating, bathing, skin care, pooping, and spitting up—showing you how you *should* be challenging some of the tried-and-true practices of taking care of an infant.

Nonetheless, it's important to understand that no single decision will make or break your child's immune system. Like everything else about babies, their immune systems are resilient. But too much damage from too many insults can cause irreversible issues. Let your goal be to foster as healthy a microbiome, barrier, and immune system as possible while also understanding that you are human, that not everything is in your control, and that a healthy child is the sum of many things.

> The habits parents put in place and the choices they make during their child's first six months can either foster strong barriers and a healthy immune system or set off a chain reaction of allergic responses that takes years to control.

. . . .

How to Bathe Your Baby

After Leo was born, my mother often stayed with us to help care for him. One night during bath time, she noted that in India, baby baths look totally different than they do in the United States. While here we put babies in a tub or basin and wash them with gentle soap, in India, babies are first massaged with coconut oil, then scrubbed with a mixture of chickpea flour and milk cream. At the end, their parents rinse them with warm water. I didn't know this at the time, but these steps are designed to enhance their skin barrier, not to clean the baby.

Since I had spent my entire life rejecting my mother's advice as outdated and foreign, I wasn't about to stop now. So I thanked her politely and promptly ignored everything she said. Then I followed all the books I'd read and washed Leo nightly using either Johnson's Baby Soap or some organic, all-natural baby bars that were supposedly better. After I dried him off, I massaged him with baby lotions. I felt happy that my baby was free of bacteria and safe, but it never occurred to me that I was stripping his skin of healthy bacteria instead of feeding it.

Leo developed red, itchy patches on his skin only a few months after he was born. When he turned six months old, the doctor diagnosed him with eczema.

Eczema is usually the first allergic disease infants develop. Preventing or even minimizing it can reduce the risk of future allergic disease by closing off pathways for food allergies and asthma to begin. As I said in chapter 1, a disrupted skin barrier allows antigens to enter the body, and that causes the immune system to go into overdrive.

Now that Leo is older, infant skin care is better studied and less controversial than it used to be, and the consensus on bathing your baby has now shifted. For the first two weeks of your baby's life, do not bathe them. Allow the vernix caseosa (the white goop covering a baby after birth) to absorb naturally. After two weeks, the American Academy of Dermatology recommends that you not bathe your baby more than three times per week.[1] However, since your infant is not a teenager with body odor headed to the prom, they really have no need for a hygiene routine. The National Health Service in the United Kingdom advises parents that there is no reason to bathe a baby for the first two to four weeks, and if you do, it recommends that you not use anything other than sterile water.[2] My research has shown me that for babies through at least six months old, baths should be given only as needed and really only with water. Before babies can crawl, they almost never get dirty. They're secure in a stroller or carrier, in your arms, or wrapped in clean diapers and clean blankets, so there's no possibility they can get into anything unsanitary.

Babies do sweat, but they do not have the bacteria that would cause them to smell. If they have blowout diapers or projectile vomit or spit-up, you will obviously want to wash them. When you do, never use harsh soaps, chemicals, or fragrance. Instead, fill a small tub or sink with three to four inches of warm water. Then use a clean washcloth to gently wipe off any food or poop. You can similarly "wash their hair" with clean warm water, and if there's anything stuck in it, you can remove it with a soft brush or comb. Gently pat your baby dry, then put them in a fresh diaper and clean clothes. That's it. That's the whole routine.

> There is no reason to bathe a baby for the first two to four weeks, and if you do, do not use anything other than sterile water.

Diaper changes are the same deal. A baby's bottom can be cleaned with gauze, cotton balls, or washcloths wet with warm water. Avoid any baby wipes with chemicals, fragrances, or soaps for at least the first month. Chemicals like methylisothiazolinone, which are commonly found in diaper wipes, can strip skin of protective microbes, disrupt natural skin pH, and cause irritation, skin breakdown, and even chemical burns.[3]

In the first few days of life, your baby's poops will be thick, dark green, sticky, and gross. Those poops are actually meconium, which is composed of everything that your baby ingested

Diaper changes are the same deal. A baby's bottom can be cleaned with gauze, cotton balls, or washcloths wet with warm water. Avoid any baby wipes with chemicals, fragrances, or soaps for at least the first month.

as a fetus, including amniotic fluid, mucus, and bile. It may feel strange to not use anything but water to wash away that gross stuff, but remember that soap is intended to dislodge germs and viruses. Your baby is drinking only pathogen-free breast milk and isn't putting their bottom on public toilet seats. You don't need to wash germs or viruses off them, but you do want to maintain and support a host of commensal bacteria in the urogenital tract, anus, and skin. After a baby's poop changes to the yellowy seeds of a breast milk diet or the yellow-brown paste of formula poop, baby wipes can be used, but they should be water only and free of alcohol or perfume.

One of the reasons my sister picked her twins' nanny was how calm and practical she was about everything. She was flexible and worked with my sister on almost every parenting decision. The one thing she wouldn't budge on, though, was using Water-Wipes, a commercial baby wipe made of only water. It seemed random to both of us at the time, but Fiona intuitively learned (after caring for forty sets of twins!) that avoiding chemical wipes made a big difference in skin integrity. England's National Health Service, along with other European pediatric guidelines, backs her up in their strong recommendation to use only water on a baby's bottom.

Diaper rash is a common concern, but you can easily avoid this if you change your baby's diaper frequently, meaning after every feeding or every one to three hours. Frequent changes will prevent ammonia buildup and avoid having fecal bacteria sit on the skin for too long. Super-absorbent diapers will keep your baby's skin dry, but more and more parents are moving to cloth diapering. I was initially skeptical, but I did it, and it's way less work than you think. Baby poop is nothing like adult or toddler poop, so it cleans off diapers with a rinse. Plus, not only is cloth diapering better for the environment and cheaper for you in the long run, but a plain cotton or bamboo layer next to your baby's skin is significantly less damaging than the chemicals that are in commercially available, super-absorbent diapers. Many cities also have cloth diapering services, but a slop sink or a washer and dryer close by will make cleaning diapers a breeze. You will be doing laundry for dirty onesies, bibs, and burp cloths almost every day anyway, so you can throw the diapers in at the same time.

If your baby does develop diaper rash, preservative-free 20 percent zinc oxide creams can help to protect and enhance the skin barrier by sealing in hydration while maintaining protective microbes. Beyond that, creams and lotions should not be used on a baby for the first couple of months unless prescribed by a pediatrician. Any cream you place on your baby's skin will be absorbed into their bloodstream, and they generally do not need it. Just leave them alone.

Based on hopeful results from some small studies, researchers thought that using emollients (non-cosmetic moisturizers that keep the skin moist and flexible) daily on a baby's skin, starting at birth, could prevent water loss and skin barrier breakdown. This would then prevent eczema. However, a large, randomized trial of 1,394 newborns concluded in 2020[4] that there was no evidence to support the idea that regular emollient use during a baby's first year reduced their risk of developing eczema. Even worse, a 2021 study showed that frequent use of emollients in children with normal skin actually increased their risk of developing allergies.[5] (Many

Creams and lotions should not be used on a baby for the first couple of months unless prescribed by a pediatrician.

doctors hypothesize that if parents don't wash their hands well of food before applying lotion, they can end up doing more damage than good.)

Later in life, you can use emollients and commercial creams like CeraVe, Cetaphil, Aquaphor, and others on your baby's skin *if needed*. Remember there's no need to unless your pediatrician recommends it for excessively dry skin. All these products are endorsed by the National Eczema Association, and critically, none of them contain foods that might trigger an allergic reaction. A number of studies have shown a link between wheat in soap, oats in skin care products, and peanut oil in moisturizers and the development of food allergies,[6] so if you must use commercial creams or lotions, stay away from anything containing food products, and always wash your hands before applying creams to your baby.

Not putting lotions on your baby's skin includes sunscreen. Instead, keep your baby out of the sun or use hats, umbrellas, and sun-protective clothing to protect their skin from ultraviolet rays. Americans have developed an obsession with sunscreen, which reduces the risk of skin cancer. However, studies have proven that the six most common active ingredients in chemical sunscreens are systemically absorbed into the blood at levels that surpass the FDA threshold at which they say a chemical is safe. With infants, there basically is no safe level of chemicals in the bloodstream.[7]

However, note that I am talking about *chemical* sunscreens, not mineral sunscreens. Chemical sunscreens penetrate the skin layers and prevent your skin cells from absorbing harmful rays. Mineral sunscreens typically contain zinc oxide and sit on the skin like a barrier. While mineral sunscreens are far safer to use than chemical ones, they are still less effective than staying out of excessive sun or wearing protective clothing.

....

Dealing with Cradle Cap

Around four months old, Leo started getting scaly whitish yellow patches of skin on his head. I didn't have to go to the internet to search for what it was; I'd seen it on my friends' babies, and I knew it was seborrheic dermatitis, commonly called cradle cap.

Or, as my friend's mother called it, cradle crap.

Unfortunately, Leo's cradle cap was flaky and itchy, and he scratched at his head in his sleep. Because babies lack motor control, and because it was impossible to keep his tiny nails trimmed, he often woke with scratches on his forehead. We tried putting mittens on his little hands, but he pulled them off at night. So we started making him wear a nightcap, but all it did was make him look like an elf.

I asked the pediatrician about Leo's cradle cap, but she—like all the baby books and websites—explained that cradle cap was normal and harmless and that I should simply ignore it. I wanted to believe her, so I tried as hard as I could, but the problem didn't get better. Leo kept scratching, and the scaly patches flaked off and started oozing angrily. Then Scott and I noticed that the intricate map of cradle cap on his head was preventing his hair from growing in.

Anyone whose baby has had cradle cap knows how unattractive it is. And while raising a baby is not a beauty contest, it was hard for us not to want to wash it off with every bath. We tried every method recommended for loosening the scaly buildup, including olive oil, baby oil, and mild shampoo, but nothing seemed to make a difference. I tried to "gently brush the excess scales" off his head (something a book suggested), but I ended up picking at some, which made them ooze more. Eventually either Leo's scratching or probably my picking caused his skin to become infected, and the pediatrician prescribed him an antibiotic to bring it under control.

Scientists believe that cradle cap is caused by an overpopulation of *Malassezia* spp. fungus on the scalp.[8] *Malassezia* eats sebum (an oily yellowish substance secreted by the aptly named sebaceous glands) and releases oleic acid, which causes excessive skin cell shedding and inflammation. It's true that in general, if the cradle cap doesn't bother your baby, you can leave it alone. But a better solution is to deal with the underlying cause: the fungus.

A better solution to cradle cap than ignoring it is to deal with the underlying cause: the fungus.

After Leo finished his course of antibiotics, I did some research and found a few clinical papers saying that anti-dandruff shampoos would reduce fungus levels and restore the scalp biome's balance. When Leo's cradle cap was especially itchy, I bought some Neutrogena T/Gel shampoo and gently washed his head with it. It smelled ridiculously chemically, and we had to be really careful not to get it in his eyes, but it got his cradle cap to subside by controlling the fungus overgrowth in one or two shampoos.

When my younger son, Kaden, developed cradle cap, we nipped it in the bud with one use of the anti-dandruff shampoo, never letting the fungus go wild or letting him scratch at his skin until it got infected. Interestingly, the same fungus that causes cradle cap is often found on children who develop eczema, and that eczema is much more severe in patients who also have *Malassezia globosa* on their skin. While I can't confirm it, sometimes I think this was another divergent point where we kept Kaden from following the same allergy-ridden path that Leo had.

....

Watching for Eczema

A week after we returned from our trip to London, when I'd first noticed how red and dry Leo's skin looked compared to that of his cousins, I shared a photo of Leo with Scott's brother. It was a casual shot we'd taken showing off a particularly funny onesie he had received as a gift.

"His elbows look really raw," Scott's brother said with what sounded like concern. "Do you think you should see the doctor about that?"

I remembered the same tone of voice coming from the owner of the baby spa my sister and I had taken our kids to, and I began to feel uncomfortable. Maybe there really *was* something wrong with Leo? I trusted my brother-in-law; he is a doctor. So at Leo's six-month appointment, I asked the pediatrician about his skin.

"I'm going to give you a referral to a pediatric allergist," she said. "I think your son has eczema."

She was the first person to use that word.

Two weeks later, Leo and I walked into an allergist's office. After we settled into a room, the allergist examined my son's skin, then confirmed that Leo had eczema. He added that because we hadn't treated the flare, his skin had become infected. Leo was prescribed a course of antibiotics to cure the infection and a steroid cream to control his eczema flare-ups. The allergist also suggested we switch from breastfeeding to a hypoallergenic formula, which is made using cow's milk that is so highly processed that any allergy-causing proteins are broken down and can be tolerated by most allergic children.

Atopic dermatitis, or eczema, is so common that about one in seven, or 14 percent, of babies develop it.[9] Eczema usually first shows up when a baby is between three and six months old, and 85 percent of eczema cases will begin during the first year of life. The timing of eczema cropping up is right on cue in terms of immune development. Around six months, the immune system is maturing, and the adaptive side is working to create antibodies necessary to tackle antigens. As you know, however, that immune response can go overboard. Around six to ten months many children begin to show the first signs of allergic conditions. Some babies clearly develop allergic issues before this window, and some do after, but this age is when a lot of parents see the immune system in action.

Eczema always begins with an itchy reddish rash. Babies will typically develop it on the face, especially the cheeks, forehead, and chin.[10] These are areas that are often wet with saliva. The second most common area to see itchy red skin is in the folds of the elbows and wrists and behind the knees. Redness in the diaper area is generally not eczema but rather diaper rash.

Many doctors will shrug at a mild eczema diagnosis, but eczema is dangerous because broken skin can easily become infected, especially if your baby scratches at it. Infections can be hard to get rid of and may require antibiotics, which can cause more allergic issues. Eczema, especially eczema infected with staph A, is also the best predictor of food allergies and asthma. In fact, the younger babies are when eczema starts appearing and the severity of their flare-ups are directly related to their risk of food allergy.[11]

Treating eczema is essentially a matter of finding your baby's eczema triggers, avoiding them, and supporting their skin barrier with emollients if it is dry or cracked. It took us a while to figure it out, but my son's triggers were non-IgE allergies to foods. That might not be the case for others. In fact, soaps are one of the most common eczema triggers. Even the "all-natural" ingredients (which are typically fruit extracts) in hand soap, shampoo, bubble bath, and body wash can irritate young skin. Household products may also contain isothiazolinone, an antibacterial, or cocamidopropyl betaine, used to thicken shampoos and lotions, and these can both irritate the skin. Detergents that remain on clothes can be another major source of skin irritation, as can wool, polyester, and dyes found in leather.

A friend of mine struggled with bad eczema on her son for months. One weekend they accidentally forgot to pack clothes for their son during a visit to friends. When his skin cleared, they realized that the change was switching from cotton/polyester blend pajamas to pure cotton ones.

Treating eczema is essentially a matter of finding your baby's eczema triggers, avoiding them, and supporting their skin barrier with emollients if it is dry or cracked.

We think of air mostly as something we breathe, but the air carries pollen and molds onto every surface in our house, including carpets, sofas, and bedsheets. Pollen in the air can trigger eczema or make it worse. So can dust mites, pet dander from cats and dogs, mold, and dandruff. To find pollen triggers, you will need to see an allergist to test your baby for environmental allergies. You can also install a strong air filtration system in your house, or smaller HEPA filters in the bedrooms, and you should dust and wash sheets frequently to remove dust mites and pollen.

A growing body of evidence shows that food allergies—often non-IgE food allergies—are at the root of eczema-like symptoms,[12] and many parents will tell you that the only way they are able to prevent their children's flares is to avoid certain foods. However, research about food allergies is constantly evolving, and all that parents need to care about is that for their child, eating a particular food will likely cause a skin flare.

The eight foods most likely to lead to allergic reactions are dairy, eggs, peanuts, tree nuts, wheat, soy, fish, and sesame. If you have a hunch that your child's eczema may be related to what they're eating—or you simply want to cross off all potential causes—eliminate these foods one by one from their diet to help identify food triggers. If you are breastfeeding, you may try avoiding allergens in your diet or simply switch to a hypoallergenic formula, as I did. An important thing to note is that non-IgE allergy symptoms can take weeks to resolve after a trigger is removed. So you will need to remove triggers for up to a month (but usually about two weeks) before attempting to reintroduce them.

> The eight foods most likely to lead to allergic reactions are dairy, eggs, peanuts, tree nuts, wheat, soy, fish, and sesame.

Lastly, given that eczema seems to develop from a combination of genetic factors and dysbiosis of the skin, something every parent can do from birth to reduce the risk of eczema is to follow the recommended healthy skin care practices given above. Maintaining healthy skin means not stripping your baby's skin of its natural oils and protective bacteria.

Breastfeeding

Few topics ignite the Mommy Wars as much as the subject of breastfeeding does, so I will say this up front: I firmly believe that a mother should do what's right for herself and her child as far as breastfeeding is concerned. While there are distinct advantages to breastfeeding in the first couple of months of a child's life, do not beat yourself up if you can't or don't. Becoming a new parent is stressful enough, so go easy on yourself.

I have been there.

Breastfeeding was easy for me at first. Both of my sons latched on right away, and my milk came in without a problem. Leo, especially, took to nursing immediately, and I thought we were both good to go when I left the hospital. At his first pediatrician visit when he was about five days old, though, the doctor mentioned something that concerned me.

"He doesn't seem to have gained any weight," she said. "While this can be normal, I want you to come back in tomorrow."

On his next visit, he still hadn't gained any weight. The next day, it was the same story.

You can't imagine the stress I felt having a child who ate all the time but didn't gain any weight. What was I doing wrong? The lactation nurse at the hospital confirmed that Leo's latch was just fine, and I assumed that since I felt a slight "rush" when Leo started feeding that I was producing enough milk. Plus, he seemed to enjoy it so much. Surely he had to be eating? But one of the problems with breastfeeding is that unless you're pumping, you will never actually know exactly how much milk you produce. So I diligently soldiered on, worried the entire time, until Leo began to pack on pounds by three weeks old.

Unfortunately, the stress didn't end there. For the rest of my six-week maternity leave, almost every time Leo nursed, he fell asleep immediately, right there in my arms. I *still* didn't know if he was getting enough milk—or getting any (after all, he was asleep!). Leo seemed happy, though, and when he put on even more weight, I forced myself to stop worrying.

On the very first day of her baby's life, a mother produces a yellow or orangish pre-milk substance called *colostrum*. When she nurses her child, the colostrum seeds the baby's gut biome with a goop of helpful nutrients, immunoglobulins, passive antibodies, and signaling peptides.[13] Interestingly, colostrum contains components of the innate and adaptive immune systems, so you could say that it provides an infant's immune foundation as well as the tools that allow it to adapt over time. All of these elements protect the newborn infant from infection and help to train and shape the emerging immune system so it can handle its environment. Colostrum also establishes beneficial bacteria in the baby's gut[14] and has a laxative effect that helps a baby produce their first poops.

Around three or four days postpartum, breast milk changes from colostrum to actual milk. Using DNA analysis, scientists have been able to estimate that primarily breastfed infants get 18.5 percent of their microbes from breast milk and an additional 5 percent from areolar (nipple) skin.[15] Unsurprisingly, they determined that babies who are primarily fed formula get 5.7 percent of their microbes from breast milk and none from the nipple itself. The contribution of bacteria from mother's milk and areolar skin is highest during the first month of life and decreases as an infant grows older. This finding fits well with other studies that show that babies who are exclusively fed pumped breast milk have a distinct gut biome from babies who are nursed.[16]

As an aside, since it's clear that a small portion of the biome comes from nipple skin, I would encourage new moms who are struggling at breastfeeding or who have chosen to exclusively bottle feed to allow their children to suckle anyway. While they may not get the same amount of breast time that a child who's nursing hours a day and throughout the night will (and believe me, hours a day is an understatement!), every little bit of microbiome seeding helps. Again, don't stress too much, but it is worth a try.

Although I was a believer in "fed is best" rather than "breast is best"—and I continue to feel this way—since delving into the role of the microbiome in allergy development, I have a new-found respect for breastfeeding. Not only does breast milk facilitate the microbial transfer that supports the development of a healthy gut biome, but it is far more beneficial than formula in terms of supporting a healthy immune system. Both a 2012 meta-analysis and a 2019 study found that supplementation with cow-milk-based formula in the *first week* can almost double the risk of a milk allergy.[17] By design, sterile formula adds no immune-regulating microbes to the infant gut. Infants are born with a lean toward Team 2 immunity (their innate immunity), but the combination of no immune-regulating microbes and an exposure to cow's milk too early can increase the risk of a cow's milk allergy.

In sum, the scientific and medical community agrees that breastfeeding in week one—and even months one and two—is ideal. But how long does breastfeeding hold first place?

The answer may surprise you.

The immune benefits of breastfeeding begin to taper off by two months postpartum once a baby starts to receive vaccinations against the most common infant illnesses. While a number of studies have shown that breastfeeding for at least six months is protective against food allergies, breastfeeding doesn't have to be exclusive *and maybe shouldn't be.* A 2020 randomized clinical trial of 500 babies proved that "daily ingestion of ≥10 mL of cow's milk formula *after one and two months* of age prevents the development of cow's milk allergy."[18] In another recent study of 1,000 healthy babies, babies fed both breast milk and formula were 61 percent less likely to develop food-protein-induced allergic proctocolitis (FPIAP), an early and common manifestation of food allergy, than those exclusively formula-fed or exclusively breastfed.[19] On the other hand, exclusive breastfeeding for at least four months was associated with lower risk of eczema. However, the effects shown were weak.[20]

The immune benefits of breastfeeding begin to taper off by two months postpartum. After that, breastfeeding doesn't have to be exclusive *and maybe shouldn't be.*

With both my sons, I felt guilty for occasionally offering them a bottle of formula in the first six months. Both boys were big eaters, though, and I couldn't always keep up while pumping at work. I traveled a lot early in their lives, and I would set alarms three times a night in my hotel rooms to pump. When I wasn't in a comfortable, private place, I pumped in airport bathrooms, the middle seat on airplanes, and the back seat of the Amtrak car, where I hoped the sound of the door between cars opening and closing would distract other passengers. When I traveled, I was often gone for three days at a stretch. I quickly realized that carrying gallons of milk through an airport, then having to unload it in front of everyone at security, was a massive headache. So I developed elaborate systems to mail milk back home overnight. But these plans sometimes fell through, so I had to add in formula.

For years, I was sure I had neglected my sons' needs in some fundamental way, but it turns out giving them formula supplementation was perhaps the only correct and protective thing I did for them.

Mothers, it's time to end the guilt. The most recent data demonstrates that breastfeeding is helpful in the beginning, but that effect rapidly diminishes. People always say that part of the reason breastfeeding is so wonderful is because it's free, but it's only free if you don't value your time. Nursing can be exhausting, stressful, painful, time-consuming—and yes, enjoyable and deeply loving—but formula feeding can give a mother freedom she desperately needs. Every mother and child is different, though, so if breastfeeding past the first two months works for you, great. But feel free to let your partner or another caretaker do the overnight feed with cow's milk formula. After six months, when your baby is exposed to different

> After six months, the *relative* importance of breastfeeding in maintaining a healthy microbiome starts to drop.

foods and environmental triggers, the *relative* importance of breastfeeding in maintaining a healthy microbiome starts to drop. In fact, supplementation may protect them from a milk allergy. Again, breastfeed for as long as it makes sense for you.

....

Pooping and Spitting Up

What goes in must come out. As any parent can tell you, what exits your baby's bottom and lands in their diaper can be solid or runny, yellow, green, brown, black, or more, smelly or odorless, and flecked with all kinds of strange and interesting objects. Pooping is a daily topic of conversation in any house with a baby, so I'll break down the process of how it happens and when you should be concerned.

As food passes through the stomach and picks up bile along the way, it becomes green. The intestines then break down the bile. Based on the capabilities of the gut microbes and the amount of time the food/bile mixture spends in the intestines, your baby's poop changes from green to yellow. As it continues to pass through the digestive tract, breaking up along the way, it eventually becomes brown. Normal poop for breastfed babies should be yellow or orange until solids are introduced, both because their gut microbes require less bile to digest breast milk and because they have fewer gut microbes to process that bile. Formula-fed babies, whose milk stays in the intestines for longer, have brown poop somewhat similar to adult poop. Once you introduce solid food, it stays in their intestines for even more time so that it can fully break down, giving their bile enough time to turn it brown.

You should always pay attention to your baby's poop color, and if it suddenly changes from the way it's supposed to look or the way it's appeared since the beginning, search for answers about what could be going on. *Occasional* green poop, blue poop, and orange poop may not be cause for alarm because it is most often caused by whatever your baby ate. For example, a baby may have poop with a bluish tinge with tiny chunks after they eat blueberries.[21] This happens because when many babies begin complementary feeding, they don't yet have the tools to fully process solid foods. If *every* meal ends up untouched or a strange color in their diaper, you may want to lay off solids for a couple of weeks and try again later. Antibiotics, medications, and other additions to the diet can also temporarily change poop color.

Bloody diarrhea, red blood in multiple stools, regular black stools with mucus, white pus in poop along with a fever, silver stools, white stools and vomiting, and red-currant-jelly poops are all causes for concern, and you should seek immediate care if your baby has one. Otherwise, poop can vary through a striking number of colors.

Beyond color, there are other things to consider. Is your baby steadily gaining weight and growing, and is your baby in any sort of pain? Babies who are eating well but not growing should give you worry because a lack of weight gain means they are not processing food correctly. Babies who spit up excessively—like Leo did—arch their backs in pain, and cry from what seems like stomach discomfort are showing obvious signs of food-protein-induced allergic proctocolitis, eosinophilic esophagitis (EoE), or food allergy. If your baby is not growing as you feel they should or if they are in persistent pain for three or more days, go see a doctor.

Diarrhea should also cause concern. I'm not talking about a runny poop on a single diaper or a day of loose stools. I mean persistent diarrhea. Diarrhea can be a sign of food allergy, EoE, irritable bowel syndrome, or many other dysfunctions. At minimum it means that the intestines are inflamed in such a way that the microbes are not processing the foods. Additionally, babies with diarrhea will lose excessive water, causing dehydration. If your baby has diarrhea for more than one day, call your doctor to investigate.

On the flip side, constipation is also a real problem. I've been there. Leo once went twelve days without pooping when he was about five months old. We brought it up to the doctor, but she didn't think it was a problem since Leo wasn't showing any signs of pain. She added that Leo must be so efficient at absorbing his breast milk that almost nothing was turning into poop.

Not all doctors agree constipation should be ignored, though. One researcher at the Children's Hospital of Philadelphia that I spoke with recently said constipation is a sure sign of chronic stress and a shutdown in the digestive system. Poop is your baby's compost, and pooping once a day is akin to regularly taking the compost out of the house. When you leave anything sitting in the colon for too long, the colon can absorb "garbage" in the same way that compost left for too long will attract flies or worse. Altering your baby's diet, adjusting your diet if you are breastfeeding, or starting a probiotic may be necessary to help balance the system so that poop moves through the chain regularly and efficiently.

I wish I had known this. After my son's pediatrician told me not to worry about his constipation, I accepted it, thinking, *Some babies just aren't meant to poop every day.* Part of me even thought I was lucky because I had fewer stinky diapers to wash than most parents. Then I started supplementing with formula, and Leo's poops became more regular. He was never what I'd call a "normal" pooper, but I reassured myself that nothing is ever truly normal when you have a new baby.

The fact is, we live in a country full of constipated people. Most people don't have enough fiber in their diet and don't drink enough water, so about half of Americans experience irregular bowel movements[22] or bowel movements that they consider unpleasant to pass. These people have babies, and they assume difficult poops are just a fact of life. Your bathroom habits also aren't exactly an accepted part of your daily conversations with friends and family, so no one talks about it. If they ask their doctor about it, constipation rarely is treated like a real medical issue. Most doctors recommend you add a fiber supplement to your diet or take a laxative when things get really rough.

I *did* talk about Leo's poops with my friends, and most people had no idea what to tell me. Coupled with my doctor's initial reassurance that everything was fine, I told myself constipation wasn't a big deal. When Leo's eczema and food allergies began, I realized I'd drive myself crazy if I had to chase down another diagnosis for his irregular poops, so I shoved the entire issue to the back of my mind.

It stayed there for six years until we changed Leo's diet and he began to poop every day. I'll talk about that more in the epilogue.

In retrospect, I should have put all the disturbing clues together and realized something serious was going on with my son—and that constipation was yet another manifestation of a dysbiotic gut. Your baby *should* be pushing all their food out through the chute with very little coming back up as spit-up. Your baby should poop every day—or most days—and the poop should pass without pain. It should be yellow if your baby has not yet been introduced to solid foods and brown if your baby is eating solids. This is the sign of a properly working gut biome, and anything else is a reason to at least investigate.

> **Your baby should poop almost every day, without pain, and have very little spit-up.**

....

Understanding Early Food Allergies

Like my son, whose symptoms were some eczema, spitting up, and some constipation, not all food allergies look the way you think. Today, most parents and even most doctors don't consider a food allergy "real" unless it shows up on an IgE blood test or it causes immediate symptoms like hives, vomiting, or trouble breathing.

But this is not exactly correct. An allergy simply means that the body is reacting to a trigger. Some allergies are caused by antibodies other than IgE, and they look very different from Macaulay Culkin's collapsing from a reaction to bee stings in *My Girl.* All kinds of allergies are serious, but some can have deadly consequences while others don't. Understanding that the strange symptoms you may see are actually allergies is critical to getting to the bottom of your child's immune illnesses. Furthermore, it will also ensure that you seek help when it's needed.

Leo, for example, always showed up as allergic to soy on testing, but he could seemingly eat soy without any kind of reaction. For years, every doctor told us to ignore this result since he wasn't reacting. Much later, after learning about mixed allergies, we eliminated soy from his diet, and like magic his eczema cleared up.

There are three types of food allergies. I'm going to call them *anaphylactic allergies, stomach allergies,* and *chronic issue allergies.* (Their scientific names are IgE-mediated, non-IgE-mediated, and mixed, respectively.) The three types of food allergies have overlaps and can be hard to tell apart, but all have some hallmark patterns.

- *Anaphylactic, or IgE-mediated, allergies* are the allergies that parents are terrified of. Anaphylactic allergies can develop at any age, but most develop in infancy when the immune system is learning. Reaction symptoms come on fast, usually within seconds or minutes of eating a food. Almost all the reactions happen within four hours, though it is possible for them to be delayed. The symptoms of anaphylactic allergies are sudden hives, redness of the skin, stomach cramping and pain, vomiting, diarrhea, coughing, sneezing, closing of the airways, and fever. Any of the symptoms above is possible, but many reactions may involve only the skin or the stomach.

  These allergies are termed IgE-mediated because the symptoms are set off by IgE antibodies. Anaphylactic allergies are diagnosed by skin-prick or blood testing because those tests measure IgE antibodies combined with a history of reactions to a food. The symptoms look like the body violently trying to eject or kill a parasite, because that's what it is doing. The reactions can stop as fast as they started if the body decides the parasite is gone.

- *Stomach, or non-IgE-mediated, allergies* are most commonly diagnosed in small babies. Because stomach allergies are reactions happening in the stomach lining, you don't tend to get the breathing issues or hives. Instead, what you see is diarrhea, watery stools, or maybe blood or mucus in stools, along with belly pain. The skin is sometimes involved, with herpes-like raised patches. The symptoms from these allergies can take days or weeks to go away even after the food is removed. Childhood stomach allergies are harder for parents to spot, and these allergies will not show up on IgE testing.

Earlier, I mentioned a group of allergies called FPIES (food-protein-induced enterocolitis syndrome), as well as enteropathy, proctitis, and proctocolitis. Different antibodies, including IgA and IgM—which are found in the mucous lining of the GI system—react to food proteins. Enterocolitis can happen anywhere in the gut, enteropathy in the small bowel, proctitis in the rectum, and proctocolitis in the colon. Symptoms from childhood stomach allergies are usually delayed four or more hours after a food is eaten, perhaps because that's how long the food can take to make its way to the reacting part of the GI system.

Technically, you can have a stomach allergy to any food, but they seem to be most common to milk, wheat, rice, oat, and other grains. By the time they are diagnosed, the baby may have been eating that food every day for weeks or months.

• *Chronic issue, or mixed IgE and non-IgE, allergies* are things like chronic eczema and eosinophilic esophagitis (EoE). As the medical name suggests, the symptoms are triggered by a combination of IgE antibodies and other immune cells, like eosinophils.

Although there is still debate on this matter, a large and growing group of doctors agree that some eczema can actually be a mixed IgE and non-IgE food allergy. The symptoms may be limited to the skin, which develops eczema patches and does not heal up with steroids. EoE is limited to issues with the esophagus, like pain when swallowing and projectile vomiting that occurs when the food can't even make it into the stomach.

Types of Food Allergy	Anaphylactic	Childhood Stomach	Chronic Issue
Doctors call it	IgE-mediated food allergy	Non-IgE-mediated allergy, aka FPIES, enteropathy, proctitis, proctocolitis	Mixed IgE and non-IgE allergy, aka atopic dermatitis and eosinophilic esophagitis
When it develops	First three years	Often in babies	Babies
Time from eating to symptoms	Seconds to four hours	Often after four hours	Feels almost unrelated to when food was eaten
Skin symptoms	Hives; also maybe redness, swelling, heat	Herpes-like patches	Chronic eczema, especially with "raw" skin
GI symptoms	Pain, vomiting, diarrhea	Diarrhea, watery stools (FPIES), or mucus or blood in stool (proctitis)	Can't swallow, projectile vomit, pain
Airway symptoms	Coughing, sneezing, tightening of airways	Not common	Not common
Time to symptoms stopping	Immediately after medication; otherwise within a few hours	Weeks, months	Weeks, months
Need EpiPen?	Yes	No	No
Treatment	Strict avoidance and immunotherapy	Remove from diet	Remove from diet

Because there are IgE cells involved in these allergies, skin-prick or blood testing will show IgE antibodies. But a lot of people have IgE antibodies without the anaphylaxis symptoms, so from there doctors should look to an elimination diet. If that food is removed and the eczema or EoE heals, and if the food is reintroduced, the eczema or EoE flares again, then you may be diagnosed with a mixed allergy.

....

Ear Infections and Other Illnesses

As I discussed in the last chapter, kids get sick a lot. Your baby will most likely develop at least one stomach bug, ear infection, cold, or other illness in their first year. This is not cause for concern. What is worth remembering, though, is that unnecessary use of antibiotics is dangerous. Make sure your doctor is following the protocol for when to use antibiotics to treat an ear infection, and when possible, ask for a prescription that you'll fill only after you determine that the infection will not clear on its own. Never use antibiotics to treat bronchiolitis, a cold, or any other illness that is viral.

Conjunctivitis, or pinkeye, is an unpleasant goopy infection that many children pick up when they start day care or school. Almost 90 percent of pinkeye is caused by a virus,[23] yet almost every baby will be prescribed an antibiotic for it. Not because they need it, but because many day care centers will demand proof of antibiotics before they let a child return. Antibiotics placed in the eye are definitely less of a concern than antibiotics that go into the gut or those are given intravenously, but they should still be avoided when possible. If you are lucky enough that the dreaded phone call from your child's day care or the school nurse comes on a Thursday or Friday, hold off on antibiotics and see if the pinkeye will resolve on its own over the weekend.

Another way parents can control how their baby is treated is to think about where they are going for the treatment. Your primary care doctor is always your best bet. Almost all doctors now have on-call services where you can speak to someone—and sometimes receive prescriptions—even when the office is closed. The COVID-19 pandemic also codified the idea of telemedicine, so now almost any doctor's office will allow you to do a video conference with a doctor from the comfort of your bed.

Try not to rush to urgent care or the emergency department for something minor like a cold, though you should definitely go if your baby is lethargic, is having trouble breathing, or is hurt. Urgent care centers are much more likely to prescribe antibiotics because—unlike your primary care doctor—they don't have the ability to check up on you or to schedule a follow-up appointment. To be on the "safe" side, they will prescribe antibiotics. I made this mistake with Kaden when he was about a year old. We panicked about a fever of 104 on a Saturday night and took him to urgent care. He was put on an antibiotic, and when his pediatrician saw him Monday morning, she said, "I wish you would have called us. He doesn't need antibiotics because they won't help for this."

The best way to avoid having to decide whether to use antibiotics is to *prevent* as many illnesses as possible. Never do the opposite and consciously let your child become sick. Since childhood illnesses stopped regularly being thought of as fatal, some parents have chosen to allow their children to contract them so they can develop the antibodies to prevent future infections. You've probably heard of chickenpox parties and playdates in the seventies and early eighties or COVID-19 parties during the pandemic. Before there were vaccines for either of these illnesses, some people decided to infect themselves or their children to "get it over with."

This might have developed antibodies, but at what cost? Willingly infecting yourself or your child can cause you to become dangerously ill and may lead to death. It's also entirely ineffective when it comes to immune diseases.

Urgent care centers are much more likely to prescribe antibiotics because—unlike your primary care doctor—they don't have the ability to check up on you or to schedule a follow-up appointment.

The hygiene hypothesis, which I discussed in chapter 1, posited that we develop allergic and autoimmune diseases because we don't get sick enough. This hypothesis has been debunked because researchers have determined that preventing common respiratory and stomach infections during infancy is not related to later development of allergic disease.[24] Instead, repeated respiratory infections can *drive* increased lung hyper-responsiveness and enhanced sensitization to allergens.[25]

In summary, there is no reason to try to get your baby sick with a cold because illness will not make their immune system stronger; it will recognize just that one cold virus. Though many supplements and home remedies claim to promote a stronger immune system, unless you have reason to believe that your baby has a persistent inability to clear infections, what you actually want is a less sensitive, less hyperactive immune system that becomes triggered only when it is absolutely needed. In short, wash your hands often and insist that all those who hold your baby also wash their hands. Definitely let your baby play in grass, dirt, and sand, but do not put them in a situation that will cause them to become sick.

....

Vaccines and the Flu Shot

Speaking of not letting your kid get sick unnecessarily, get them vaccinated. We have vaccines to prevent diseases that have killed millions of people, including over half of my aunts and uncles. The worst part is that those who have died from these avoidable diseases were most often children. Thankfully, since the advent of vaccines, mortality for children under five has dropped considerably.

Instead of having to get really sick in order to learn how to fight an infection, vaccines teach your immune system to fight specific pathogens so that if you encounter that pathogen in the future, your body will be able to recognize and squash it quickly and effectively.

Vaccines are made of either a dead version of the pathogen (inactivated), a living but weakened version of the pathogen (attenuated), a piece of the pathogen (subunit), or DNA/RNA from the pathogen (nucleic acid). Recall the analogy that our immune system is like a chaotic airport. Before bad guys show up at the airport, vaccines teach the airport security to recognize those bad guys and kick them out. Vaccines show the airport security a corpse of a bad guy, a handcuffed bad guy, a bad guy's unique tattoo, or instructions on how to bring the bad guy down. Inactivated, attenuated, and subunit vaccines give the airport security a chance to practice and to learn how to kick out a bad guy. DNA/RNA vaccines simply pass on the instructions for how to win.

Live, attenuated viruses (handcuffed)—such as the smallpox vaccine—often provide lifelong immunity, but they are not always appropriate for people with compromised immune systems who cannot fight off even a weak enemy. Inactivated vaccines (corpses) are safer, but they are more difficult to make, and most people require periodic boosters. These include the flu and polio vaccines. Subunit vaccines (tattoos)—such as hepatitis B and shingles—work well, with a long memory, and are considered even safer. Until the COVID-19 pandemic, DNA/RNA vaccines were hard to make. But drug companies did the impossible and created mRNA COVID-19 vaccines within a year. The mRNA vaccines are considered the safest of all, because none of the actual virus is in the vaccine, just instructions for beating the virus. Now that we are better at making DNA/RNA vaccines, look for a massive switchover to them.

It's important that you understand this. No matter which way the vaccine version of the pathogen is presented—attenuated, inactivated, subunit, or DNA/RNA—the immune system develops defenses against the specific pathogen it is shown and nothing else. And with each passing year, vaccines get better and more specific. Decades ago, vaccines used to include many more antigens (think of them like examples) for the immune system to learn what it needed. As we have discovered which antigens are most effective, we have reduced the number of antigens in each vaccine. Children today are actually receiving fewer and more targeted vaccines than children a generation ago.

Here's why infant vaccines are critical. The vaccines that are part of the infant vaccination schedule protect against bacteria and viruses that commonly infect children. Hepatitis B, diphtheria, tetanus, pertussis, *Haemophilus influenzae* type b infection, pneumococcal disease, polio, rotavirus, and flu are particularly dangerous diseases for babies. A pertussis infection that an adult might easily recover from can be deadly to an infant.

Babies are born with some immunity passed to them from their mother while they are in utero and through breast milk.

However, newborns—whose immune systems are very much in development—lack much adaptive immunity, which is the ability to respond effectively to infections. That is why babies are at much higher risk from infections and why doctors do not wait and see as much before giving antibiotics to children under age two. This is also why vaccines against illnesses are so important for babies.

You may have heard that vaccines may cause allergies or autism. This theory has been definitively debunked, and today the science is clear: vaccines are not harmful, and there is simply no reason to avoid them. Here's why you should not worry about vaccines and immune diseases. (After all, this whole book is about reducing the risk of immune disease. If there was evidence they were linked, I would say so!)

The first reason you can feel comfortable that infant vaccines do not cause allergic disease is that vaccines activate different teams (Team 1 and Team 17) from the team that overreacts in allergic diseases (Team 2). If you don't fully remember the lesson on T helper cells, or as we called them, Teams 1, 2, and 17, don't worry. All you need to know is that each Team—1, 2, and 17—responds to viruses, parasites, and bacteria, respectively. A vaccine for a bacterium or virus will teach Team 1 and Team 17 to respond quickly but will have little effect on Team 2. Bacterial vaccines will not cause Team 2 cells to do much of anything because that's not Team 2's job.

The second reason we know vaccines don't cause immune disease is that they elicit a pretty small immune response, especially relative to the actual disease. In fact, many vaccines contain adjuvants (chemical substances that boost the effectiveness of a vaccine), like alum in the Hep B vaccine, to make sure that the immune system recognizes the vaccine and doesn't completely ignore it. The few adjuvants, like alum, which are known to have a small Team 2 response, have been studied, and no link has been found between the Hep B vaccine and allergies.

Vaccines also stimulate the immune system for a very limited time. When a pathogen enters the body—even when in vaccine form—the immune system reacts immediately. The immune system stops reacting once it has effectively fought and cleared the pathogen and developed antibodies. Once the pathogen is gone, the immune system returns to its original state.

Is combining vaccines safe? Yes. The reason we can combine them is that vaccines have gotten better and more specific over the years. In terms of teaching the body to fight off bad guys, the subunit and DNA/RNA vaccines are as effective but way more specific, meaning they use a smaller immune response for the same amount of protection. As we learn which tattoo, or subunit, is the most effective identifier of a particular pathogen bad guy, we are making vaccines more specific and reducing the number of antigens they use. As said before, though it's counterintuitive, many of the combined vaccines today have fewer total antigens and therefore stimulate the immune system less than their individual versions a generation ago.

The third reason we can trust that vaccines are safe is that even when they have additives like MSG and gelatin that could cause allergic reactions, such responses are incredibly rare. MSG and gelatin are preservatives used to make vaccines resilient to heat or cold. Gelatin in vaccines causes about one case of anaphylaxis for every two million injections. This is a tiny risk, and notably, none of the top eight food allergies are in vaccines.

However, I think the most convincing proof that vaccines don't cause food allergies is that vaccine schedules are very consistent across Western countries, while food allergy rates are not. For example, Germany and Israel have the same vaccine schedule as the United States but drastically lower food allergies. It's

Vaccine	Birth	1 mo	2 mos	4 mos	6 mos	9 mos	12 mos	15 mos
Hepatitis B (Hep B)	1st dose	2nd dose					3rd dose	
Rotavirus (RV) RV1 (2-dose series); RV5 (3-dose series)			1st dose	2nd dose				
Diphtheria, tetanus, and acellular pertussis (DTaP: <7 yrs)			1st dose	2nd dose	3rd dose			4th dose
Haemophilus influenzae type b (Hib)			1st dose	2nd dose			3rd or 4th dose	
Pneumococcal conjugate (PCV13)			1st dose	2nd dose	3rd dose		4th dose	
Inactivated poliovirus (IPV: <18 yrs)			1st dose	2nd dose			3rd dose	
Influenza (IIV)						Annual vaccination 1 or 2 doses		

far more likely that all the other environmental and dietary differences between countries are the cause of immune disease.

....

Your Options When It Comes to Vaccines

I spoke with Dr. James R. Baker Jr., director of the Mary H. Weiser Food Allergy Center at the University of Michigan, at length about vaccines and allergic disease. He assured me that his vaccine research lab spends considerable time—and has received significant funding—to look critically at issues of vaccine design or timing. For example, in the past it has suggested delaying some vaccines or using different adjuvants that have a smaller Team 2 response, such as RNA vaccines.

"But changing the process of administering vaccines has to be weighed against different factors," he added. "The reason we give hepatitis B at birth is because the most common way people get hepatitis B is *during* birth. In Asia, where the rates of hepatitis B are much higher than here, many children can wind up with hepatoma [a tumor of the liver that is usually malignant]. So we certainly don't want to delay the vaccine in Asia. The trade-off wouldn't make sense."

While protecting the advances we have made against a number of diseases, we can simultaneously continue to improve vaccines. The pneumococcal vaccine—which works to prevent some types of pneumonia, sepsis, and meningitis—reduces the number of pneumococcal bacteria in infants. This is a good and bad thing; pneumococcus can cause deadly infections, but it is also a normal part of our microbiome. In the same way that treating *Helicobacter pylori* stopped stomach ulcers but possibly caused an increase in reflux disease, more research should and will be done on how losing pneumococcus affects the broader microbiome.

In addition, a more relaxed vaccine schedule is also acceptable as long as children get their vaccines before school. A different schedule might allow parents to avoid introducing new foods two to four weeks after a vaccination or delay the six-month vaccinations to nine or twelve months, when they've introduced all the common foods and triggers in their environment. There's nothing necessarily wrong with a slower schedule. The reason that the CDC follows the current schedule is that parents are already at the doctor's office for well visits. Adding more visits is hard on many families and can lead to missed vaccines. Most

doctors will work with you as long as your child can be vaccinated before they are in high-exposure situations, like school,
on a regular basis.

Lastly, we know that immunocompromised people cannot
receive live attenuated vaccines because their immune systems
are not strong enough to handle them. The MMR (measles,
mumps, rubella), rotavirus, and chickenpox vaccines are all attenuated and part of the normal infant immunization schedule.
Given that a large percentage of infants today have an abnormal
immune system caused by dysbiosis, we should do more research
on how vaccines are being tolerated. Especially with the likely
move to RNA vaccines, it's a good time to understand if vaccines
can exacerbate already existing immune issues in infants and
what can be done to maintain our gains against deadly childhood
diseases.

....

In Conclusion

The first six months of your child's life are about respecting their
microbiome as much as possible and nipping as many issues in
the bud as possible. I so wish Scott and I had known this. When
we failed to take Leo's eczema seriously early on, we practically
led him along the allergic or atopic march (the natural progres-
sion of allergic diseases). It took us months to get to anything
resembling a stable routine, and every couple of weeks it seemed
like he developed a new issue or the same issue in a different
spot. We would seek help from his doctors, and his care regimen
would change. The changes were so fast and furious that my
husband started making Google Docs titled "L Care Week of . . ."
One week Leo was using an antifungal cream at eleven A.M. and
seven P.M. A couple of weeks later, we switched creams and added

in antibiotics and steroids at three P.M. Then we began giving Leo bleach baths at night and a hypoallergenic formula all throughout the day. There was less nursing with more formula one week and more nursing with less formula the next. We bought new detergents, different sheets, new diapers, and on and on and on.

Proactively caring for the microbiome and identifying problems early can prevent conditions from spinning out of control. For most babies, that means doing *less work*. Bathe your baby less often with fewer chemicals. Protect their skin with fewer products and cover them with hats and clothes rather than sunscreen. Breastfeed in the beginning, but don't stress about adding formula after a month. Use what you have at your disposal between good bathing practices, emollients, antifungal shampoos, and diet changes to stop itchy red patches, and encourage a daily, pain-free poop. Finally, take them to the doctor only when it's really needed.

> **Proactively caring for the microbiome and identifying problems early can prevent conditions from spinning out of control.**

But if your instincts are telling you something is off, listen. You are your child's caregiver and protector, and you should never stop striving to get to the bottom of a problem.

....

CHAPTER FIVE

The Importance
of a Good Diet

Common Misconception:
An occasional little bit of
added sugar won't hurt your child.

....

Children under the age of two should have *no* added sugar
(meaning white sugar, honey, syrup, sucrose, high-fructose corn
syrup, and more) or artificial sweeteners. High-fructose corn syrup
(HFCS) and aspartame have been shown to be toxic to gut bacteria. HFCS in high doses can also disrupt the gut biome, and
therefore the gut lining, causing leaky gut syndrome.

Leo was six pounds when he was born, which is small but not
concerning for an infant. He started to pack on weight a few
weeks after he was born, and since he was three months old, he's
been big for his age. He loved every bottle or breastfeeding ses-
sion, and I often struggled to keep up with how much milk he

needed. By the time he was four months old, he was reaching for the solid food he'd see on our plates. But we held off letting him try anything because every book we'd read and every parent or doctor we had talked to said we should give him only breast milk or formula until he was six months old.

Right at six months, we started by giving Leo pureed peas. Then we followed the prevailing advice—that has zero scientific backing—to introduce only one new food every three days. We diligently avoided eggs, dairy, nuts, and soy products—the most common childhood food allergy triggers—because that's what everyone said to do. When Leo had advanced through the "new food every three days" introduction process we incorrectly thought we were supposed to do, we began pureeing whatever we were having for dinner and feeding it to him with a spoon.

Being nervous new parents, we briefly wondered if purees were not the way to go. The hot new trend was baby-led weaning, a process where parents offer their babies finger foods and let them feed themselves. We tried it a couple of times, but it was incredibly messy, actually required more prep work than the homemade purees, and didn't really free us up because we had to keep helping him pick up the pieces. For a big eater, gnawing on chunks of food led to a lot of frustration and crying when he couldn't eat enough. Plus, he ate most of his meals at day care. It just didn't work for us.

Leo ate every kind of food, and to this day, he loves rich, complex flavors. For lunches and dinners, we pureed or chopped up curries, rice dishes, salads, pastas, and even uncommon vegetables like Jerusalem artichokes. But babies need to eat five or six times a day, and when we weren't eating with him, it seemed silly to cook a whole other meal. That's how the snacks crept in, one by one. In the moment, snacks felt like a tiny, harmless part of his diet, but in truth, these non-nutritious snacks contained added sugar, and that sugar eventually made up a significant portion of his overall calories.

I'm guessing that last paragraph about snacks probably made you a little bit anxious. Talking about a healthy diet is where many motivated folks throw their hands in the air. Feeding your children well day in and day out is generally not convenient and is certainly more time-consuming, and once your kids are used to added sugar, a healthy diet seems less tasty to them. Seeing children rejecting healthy food often becomes a painful battle of wills, and few of us want our dinner table to be a war zone dominated by a tiny tyrant who is having a tantrum. However, we are going to talk about a healthy diet anyway because it is vitally important. Immune diseases are clearly related to the health of our gut microbiome, and what babies eat from their first bites matters. Most of the advice in this chapter won't be new to you. But I'm going to explain why it's true because understanding diet's link to the biome and the barriers will make the effort of turning mealtime around worth it.

....

Starting Solids

Between four and six months old, most babies are ready to eat solid food. The classic clues that they are ready include the ability to hold their head steady (they need strong neck muscles to swallow) and the ability to sit with support (because you can't eat lying down).

For a baby's first year, eating solids is referred to as *complementary feeding* because all their nutritional needs are met with breast milk or formula. The solid foods a baby eats are mostly intended to get them accustomed to foods' tastes and textures and to develop their chewing muscles and hand-eye coordination.

There is no need to expose babies to solids before they are ready. On the flip side, there is no need to wait until they are six months old. As early as four months is fine, but introducing solids before sixteen weeks can increase your child's risk of developing food allergy because a baby's system is not ready.[1] Never add baby cereal or other food to their bottle. It will cause your child to drink less milk or formula and not receive the essential nutrients they need.

When your baby is ready for complementary feeding, the single most important thing you can do for their immune system is to expose them to a wide variety of healthy foods in a baby-safe way. A recent study showed that babies who ate from every food group—starchy and non-starchy vegetables, fruit, meat, dairy, seeds, nuts, fish, and grains—had almost no food allergies. The more food groups they were exposed to, the fewer the allergies.

There is no need to expose babies to solids before they are ready. Anytime between four and six months is fine.

To get all these different foods in, you can puree the food, cut it into grabbable pieces, or whatever is easiest. In her book *Inventing Baby Food: Taste, Health, and the Industrialization of the American Diet*, Amy Bentley describes how what is "best" for babies goes through cycles. Sometimes parents and doctors swear by purees because they allow you to feed your child a wide variety of foods without the fear of choking. At other times, the consensus switches, saying baby-led weaning is the best way to introduce solids. Later everyone swears by nutrient-dense purified smoothies. The truth is that babies have continued to thrive throughout all these trends, so it probably doesn't matter which you choose.

As you look for what works best, you may also want to consider a feeding method practiced throughout the world but forgotten in Western countries. Before blenders and Gerber baby food was common in households, mothers would chew tough foods into a soft puree-like texture and feed it to their babies. In this way, parents could feed their baby anything that was on the dinner table.

I know this may sound a little crazy or disgusting, but bear with me. There are two real benefits to this practice. The first is that you don't have to carry baby food around with you all the time. A baby can eat almost anything you eat as long as you sufficiently grind it up with your teeth. Second, as you chew, your saliva mixes into the food. What is saliva full of? Your oral bacteria, which are a large component of your gut bacteria. As long as you have clean, healthy teeth and gums, passing your child your beneficial bacteria is like adding a probiotic to their food.

....

Early Allergen Introduction

After diet diversity, the next most important practice for developing a healthy, disease-free immune system is to give your baby regular exposure to the most common food allergens, which are nuts, eggs, dairy, wheat, sesame, and soy. Regularly means one to two times a week, making sure your child gets about two grams of the protein per serving. Different forms of food will have more or less protein. The focus here is on getting enough of the protein from each food.

This recommendation may come as a

> After diet diversity, the next most important practice for developing a healthy, disease-free immune system is to give your baby regular exposure to the most common food allergens.

surprise if you had a child before 2015, as I did. Back then, pediatricians suggested that infants *not* be given allergens until they were one, two, or even three years old. Clear clinical data now supports the idea that early introduction is critical to preventing food allergies.[2]

Much of the science on immune disease is still in the laboratory and exploratory research stage. Only a few treatments or practices have moved over to clinical research in humans. Food allergy prevention is one area where it has. Starting with the LEAP study and followed by the 2016 Enquiring About Tolerance (EAT) study, the 2014 PETIT study (whose name is too long to mention), and the 2018 CHILD study (same), these four independently run, randomized clinical trials have proven that we can prevent the immune mistakes that result in a food allergy by *feeding children those foods regularly during complementary feeding.* The studies together enrolled thousands of babies across multiple countries. Half the babies ate allergens during complementary feeding, while half avoided them. The babies who ate allergens regularly had 65 to 80 percent fewer food allergies.

To be clear, food allergies were prevented only if babies consumed the foods regularly. If the babies didn't eat at least one serving of two grams of each protein every week, they were just as likely to develop food allergies as babies who avoided the foods.[3]

With this book, one of my main goals is to focus on interventions or strategies that have the most benefit—and ideally involve the least effort. Early allergen introduction is one of them. I missed the boat on it with Leo, but when Kaden was born, I made sure to do it right. He came into the world nine months after we learned of Leo's food allergies, and my dozens of hours of research taught me to give him these foods early on.

I need to be honest here. When I began complementary feeding and early allergen introduction with Kaden, I really struggled. I bought every major allergen and spent dozens of hours figuring out how to get each food into a baby-safe form without adding any salt, sugar, or junk. I also placed Kaden's food on one side of the counter and Leo's on another so I could be positive that there wouldn't be any cross contamination. Almost every day I made two meals for two boys at the same time I had a demanding full-time job, a pumping schedule, and a husband I wanted to talk to more than a few minutes a day.

I knew there had to be a better way.

In June 2017 I took everything I had learned and started my company, Lil Mixins, to give parents the education and tools to easily introduce early allergens into their baby's meals. I did not write this book to sell my products, but I do want you to know that there are companies, websites, and resources like mine that will help make early allergen introduction seamless. You don't have to make two meals on two different sides of your kitchen. You don't even need to rush out to the store to buy every tree nut and the best kind of mortar and pestle to grind nuts into a baby-safe form. There are better and easier ways that won't drive you crazy.

But as Dr. Carina Venter, coauthor of the American Academy of Allergy, Asthma, and Immunology's 2020 guidelines on food allergy prevention,[4] says, "The most important message is to introduce all food allergens from the time your baby starts solids and keep them in your baby's diet regularly, taking your family's food patterns into account." As a registered dietitian, she understands that what works for each family is going to be different, but the goal is the same.

THE THEORIES BEHIND EARLY ALLERGEN INTRODUCTION

Looking again at the microbiome can help explain the magic of early allergen introduction. The dual-exposure hypothesis says that when food proteins cross the skin barrier, it triggers an immune response rather than immune tolerance. This immune response is heightened if a baby's skin is cracked (allowing allergens to penetrate deeply) and especially if their skin is dysbiotic (like a staph infection also triggering the immune system). When a baby eats food, though, their gut microbiome sends immune-*regulating* signals. Food protein is everywhere in a household, and babies encounter it as they roll and crawl. If a baby is exposed to food only on their skin, but not through their gut, their immune system becomes sensitized. If you give your baby food during the same period that they encounter it on their skin, they can properly regulate against unnecessary sensitization.

Another emerging explanation focuses on the infant gut biome and gut barrier. You may recall that numerous studies have shown that babies who develop food allergies have different gut biomes from babies who don't. The clearest was the study of babies in Finland and Russia, which showed that Finnish babies were missing bacteria that built up their gut barrier with protective mucus and were also missing species that signaled the body to produce Treg cells, which calm the immune system down.[5]

Both skin health and gut health are often dependent on diet. No matter which hypothesis is more correct, we know that as a baby increases the amount of solid food they eat, their diet begins to serve a primary role in shaping their microbiome. Unfortunately, a diet of sugary pureed fruit, artificially sweetened yogurt pouches, and sweetened baby cereal does everything *but* support it.

DIET BECOMES HEALTH

The idea that what your baby eats influences how their biome develops isn't just anecdotal; it's backed by research. A 2014 study comparing Italian and African children's gut microbiomes showed that after the introduction of solid foods, a significant diet-related shift occurred.[6] Before weaning, all the babies had similar gut biomes. During and after weaning, the biomes were more determined by what they ate. This suggests that when babies stop exclusively drinking breast milk, their gut bacteria are no longer determined by the breast milk.

It's worth taking the time to think through this transition. If the gut bacteria are fed by whatever food you give them, it makes sense that if you change what you eat, your gut biome will change as well. Some foods you consume can also be toxic to some types of bacteria. There is no "good" or "bad" gut biome in the moral sense. But certain types of bacteria thrive in the presence of fibrous vegetables and lead to better health, and other types flourish on sugar and will do you no good.

One clear pathway elucidated by Dr. Caroline Roduit, a pediatric allergy and immunology specialist, and her research team in Zurich is that when babies eat a diet that is high in fruits and vegetables, they have increased levels of specific bifidobacteria and lactobacilli.[7] The bacteria create a short-chain fatty acid called butyrate as they eat fiber indigestible to humans. Butyrate directly increases a baby's levels of regulatory cells and prevents allergic disease.

If a good diet is about creating good health, though, we need to pause and agree on what health *is*. Most of us have no idea what it means for our babies to be healthy. We worry about whether they meet certain developmental benchmarks like reaching for objects or crawling, and we may anxiously compare notes with friends about how many words they utter by a year. With our doctors, we focus on height and weight growth charts, learning whether our children are growing "as they should be." The truth is that developmental milestones can be fluid, and growth charts are useless measures of true health.

Good health actually means being able to sleep well through the night around six months or so, poop daily, experience minimal gas or tummy pain, and resist sickness. A healthy child should have clear skin that doesn't itch and has no rough patches or rashes, and they should be bright-eyed and alert, without eye circles or puffiness. A well child should have energy, not too many tantrums, and the ability to focus on games or toys and play with others. This is the true definition of a thriving child.

None of the "healthy" definitions above should be qualified with "when using inhalers, steroids, and drugs."

Today, far too many children are unhealthy. A generation or two ago, almost every parent could expect that their baby would be well because a healthy diet was the default. Issues like constipation, irritable bowel syndrome (IBS), type 2 diabetes, and more were simply unheard of in children. Unfortunately, with today's food system and environment, you are going to have to work against the grain (literally!) and fight hard to provide a healthy diet to your child. In fact, it's such a challenge that you must spend as much energy thinking about what *not* to do as what you should do.

AVOID SUGAR AND SWEETENERS

Your easiest and most important gut-promoting dietary priority is to avoid added sugar—especially artificial sweetener—in your baby's food. Some of the most pathogenic bacteria and fungi that can exist in your microbiome thrive on sugar. Diets high in sugar also completely throw off a body's insulin production, causing an increase in cholesterol, adipose (fat) tissue, and more.

Your easiest and most important gut-promoting dietary priority is to avoid added sugar—especially artificial sweetener—in your baby's food.

In 1800, the average person consumed 22.4 grams of sugar each day. By 1900, sugar consumption had risen to 112 grams per day. Today, Americans on average consume 227 grams of sugar each day.[8] This tenfold increase in sugar intake has had profound effects on health, including across-the-board increases in cardiovascular disease, obesity, type 2 diabetes, certain cancers, kidney failure, nonalcoholic fatty liver disease, and cognitive decline.

If those conditions occur primarily in adults, just imagine what's happening to our children, whose developing systems are far more vulnerable.

Good dietary habits begin early. That's why the American Heart Association says that children under age two should have *no added sugar* in their diets,[9] while children up to age eighteen can consume up to 25 grams of sugar *per day*. For comparison, one can of Coca-Cola has 39 grams of sugar in it. Added sugar includes any white sugar, honey, maple syrup, sucrose, high-fructose corn syrup, and more. Added sugar does not include fructose (the sugar naturally occurring in fruit) and lactose (the sugar naturally occurring in milk).

Sugar is incredibly addictive, even more so for children, who prefer their food two to three times as sweet as adults do. Any book or article you read on the topic of sugar will remind you that, in lab tests, rats will work themselves to death in search of the sweet taste of saccharin before they do the same for cocaine.[10] We are hardwired to prefer sugary foods because when sugar was not easy to come by, a sweet food meant calories that would keep our energy high and our bellies satisfied.

Today, sugar means the exact opposite. Instead of something to satisfy an energy need quickly, it's pretty much a lethal drug.

In babies and toddlers, sugar almost always replaces high-fiber foods. Think about it. How many times have you grabbed a quick ice cream as a treat or packed your child's lunch box with "fruit snacks" (which are basically gummy bears with less sugar) rather than high-fiber foods like nuts, apples, and even popcorn? When your kid wants something sweet, cut-up fruit, in its natural fibrous form, is the way to go. Cut-up cheese, olives, bell peppers, carrots, and cucumbers will also go down easy with some peanut butter or sunflower butter.

The more sugar children eat, the less likely they are to enjoy the flavor of high-fiber foods. As pediatric nutritionist Jill Castle told me in an interview for this book, "Sugar in food crowds out actual nutrients." Babies who eat sugar do not get the iron and other nutrients that build their brain scaffold, their barriers, and their microbiome.

Sugar can come in many forms, but for babies and toddlers, the most pernicious varieties are fruit concentrates in food and high-fructose corn syrup in snacks, juice or fruit drinks, candy, and breakfast cereal. Children should only rarely—meaning less than once a week—have juice (stripped of all fiber), and only if it is 100 percent fruit juice. Toddlers should never drink soda, sip a flavored coffee, or consume sports drinks. In the United States, sugar is an ingredient in almost *every* packaged food. (In years of searching, I have found only one presliced bread sold in grocery stores—Heidelberg brand—that didn't contain sugar. And you can buy it only in the Catskills.) Truly avoiding sugar means shopping, cooking, and eating from the produce, dairy, butcher, and fish aisles only.

Fructose in fruit is an acceptable form of sugar when eaten as a whole food with the fiber and skin. Obviously, there are some fruits that can't be eaten with the skin, such as mangoes. Be careful with these. While fruits such as oranges and mangoes are high in fiber and relatively low in calories—surprising given how sweet they taste—they are also full of fructose. Babies should avoid eating too many pouched baby foods made primarily with fruit because the pulp extraction process removes all the fiber. Most baby pouches that claim to be "spinach and pear" are really 90 percent pear and 10 percent spinach and strained of all fiber. Because baby food manufacturers (even the most ethical ones) want babies to suck down their foods and not waste any, almost all such pouches are designed to be sweet. Though this is okay in theory, in practice it makes babies far less willing to eat anything other than sickly sweet food.

The worst versions of sugar are artificial sweeteners. Substances like saccharin, sucralose, and aspartame were supposed to offer us all the benefits of sweetness with none of the side effects of sugar. In reality, these substances have been shown to be toxic to gut bacteria.[11] High-fructose corn syrup, which is found in everything from sodas to baked goods to catsup, can—in high doses—disrupt the gut lining, causing leaky gut syndrome, which means cracks in the lining of the intestines that cause inflammation.[12] In adults, aspartame is proven to cause irritable moods, depression, and dizziness, even when consumed at levels below the accepted maximums.[13] High-fructose corn syrup, aspartame, and other artificial sweeteners are incredibly dangerous, and I will go so far as to say that they should be avoided at all costs—especially for babies and toddlers.

Stevia is a natural sugar substitute that comes from a plant related to chrysanthemums and native to South America. Stevia is 30 to 150 times sweeter than sugar, so you can add a tiny amount to foods and find that it has the same sweetening effect as a teaspoon of sugar. Don't be fooled by the claims

The worst versions of sugar are artificial sweeteners.

that stevia is "natural," though. Many commercial sweeteners that have stevia as their base also contain a host of other ingredients rather than only pure stevia leaf. One of these ingredients may be sugar alcohols, which can cause bloating and digestive upset.

A 2020 study published in *Molecules* also showed that stevia may be as harmful to the gut biome as artificial sweeteners.[14] The bacteria in the gut have established communication pathways that allow them to regulate their levels. The presence of stevia may interrupt these pathways, disrupting the gut not by killing bacteria but by inhibiting their ability to communicate. So steer clear of stevia. It's just not worth it for a tiny bit of momentary pleasure.

The conclusion here is pretty obvious. There should be no added sugar in your child's diet before the age of two. A good rule of thumb is to keep natural sugar to less than 10 percent of their diet and be judicious about what you give them, because the sweeter foods are, the more they'll crave them. Never give babies and toddlers sugary drinks, and avoid artificial sweeteners like they are poison—because they are. Finally, think hard about what you're putting in your child's body. We are bombarded day in and day out with toxins we don't fully understand and can't necessarily measure. Why would you want to add to that by knowingly putting junk on your child's plate?

AVOID FOODS CONTAINING TOXINS, DYES, AND PESTICIDES

Toxins are everywhere in the American diet. Processed foods contain poisons in the form of preservatives, dyes, synthetic fats, and emulsifying agents, while nonorganic fruits and vegetables and factory farmed meats are full of glyphosate (an herbicide commonly known as Roundup), antibiotics, pesticides, and even plastic. Some of these chemicals, like emulsifiers, are directly poisonous to your gut barrier because they damage the bonds between the epithelial cells of the gut, while others are toxic for your commensal gut bacteria.

You may be surprised to hear that every country in Europe forbids these additives across the board, in *all* their foods. Europeans don't have to shop in the organic section of the produce aisle. *Everything* is organic. Europe follows a precautionary principle; it doesn't allow a substance to enter the food system unless it has been proven safe. In the United States, we take the opposite route. We add things, then remove them after they've caused damage—and only if scientists (who are persistently underfunded by the government) can prove that they caused harm.

This was the case with four types of red dye in the 1950s, 1960s, and 1970s. Despite the fact that food manufacturers swore these food additives had been rigorously tested and determined to be safe, the Food and Drug Administration (FDA) banned red dyes 1, 2, 4, and 32 because they were proven to cause organ damage and cancer. Mind you, this was after people had been ingesting them for *years.*

The bigger problem is that even after an ingredient has been determined to be harmful—like the antibiotics added to animal feed or the glyphosate used in grains—it's complicated and difficult to eliminate the use of them, pass regulations against them, and take them out of circulation. It's difficult to regulate the amount that is put into food, too. Kids love brightly colored foods, rainbow pancakes, and sprinkles on everything. Yet almost all the dyes that go into food have not been studied specifically considering the infant and toddler brain, their microbiomes and barriers, or their immune systems. Nor have these additives been sufficiently tested for safety or to establish levels at which they become dangerous. At doses of more than 10 milligrams, tartrazine, or yellow 5, was shown to affect children's behavior, causing them to be irritable, restless, and have trouble sleeping.[15] A single juice box can have up to 50 milligrams of dyes, including yellow 5.

Dyes can be more pernicious when combined with preservatives, too. A double-blind placebo-controlled study looked at nearly 2,000 three-year-olds who were fed a diet that contained yellow 5 and benzoate, then given a diet without those additives. At the times their diets contained yellow 5 and benzoate, parents said their children showed "significantly greater increases in hyperactive behavior." Because of studies like this, countries in Europe banned all synthetic dyes from baby food, and some went as far as to ban it in food marketed to children.

What's most upsetting is that food manufacturers *did* remove dyes and preservatives from European foods, but they kept the dyes and preservatives *in the equivalent brands sold in the United States.* Apparently unless it is specifically forbidden, proven toxins are considered safe here. For that reason, this former lover of Jell-O and rainbow cupcakes has now banned them from our house. I didn't consent for my kids to be part of a "wait and see if a problem develops" study.

Today, Scott and I try to buy organic food for our family when it makes sense practically and financially. One of the reasons to eat organic is that it encourages farms to grow healthier crops on better-maintained soil, with more rotation. Without the use of fertilizers and pesticides, it is not possible to grow the exact same crops every year on the exact same fields. The other reason is simply to reduce the amount of pesticide that you—and your children—consume. Apples, bell peppers, celery, grapes, hot peppers, peaches, pears, nectarines, spinach, strawberries, and tomatoes are called the "Dirty Dozen"[16] because they retain the highest levels of pesticides after harvesting. These fruits and vegetables should be avoided if you cannot buy them organic, but if that's not an option for you, perhaps opt for frozen versions or locally grown ones, or wash and peel them.

On the other hand, the "Clean Fifteen"[17]—avocados, sweet corn, pineapple, onions, papaya, frozen sweet peas, asparagus, eggplant, cauliflower, cantaloupe, broccoli, mushrooms, cabbage, honeydew, and kiwis—all have minimal levels of pesticides if purchased from the nonorganic section.

What about GMO (genetically modified) foods? This is a tricky subject because these foods are very poorly studied. Many people think GMO means simply plants whose DNA has been actively changed with genes from other plants or bacteria. However, we have been crossbreeding plants for hundreds of years— which is effectively swapping DNA—meaning that the foods that come from them are genetically modified, too. A peach from several thousand years ago would be unrecognizable today. What few studies are done these days on GMO plants don't clarify what kind of modification they are talking about. Therefore, while it's possible that the way your body processes plants with "alien" DNA is different, in truth we simply don't know. It would take years or decades to uncover trends, and by then the plants may have been modified multiple times. There is no good data on GMO foods, so I withhold any recommendations.

I believe the bigger concern with GMO plants is that they are often developed specifically to withstand large doses of fertilizers or chemicals that not only stay on the plants but wash into waterways and hurt farmworkers. Weeds and pests will always become pesticide resistant, requiring an arms race of ever more pesticide to keep the bugs away.

We cannot handle any more pesticides in our bodies, and it is especially urgent for our children. Glyphosate, also known as Roundup, is used extensively in growing industrial grain. Glyphosate was classified as a "probable human carcinogen" in 2015 by the International Agency for Research on Cancer, part of the World Health Organization. Since then, Bayer has paid billions[18] to settle claims that glyphosate causes cancer. Beyond cancer, though, glyphosate has been shown to cause reproductive issues such as infertility, miscarriages, birth defects, and an inflammatory bowel disease virtually indistinguishable from celiac disease.[19]

Almost all the nonorganic wheat, oat, rye, and barley on the market is soaked in glyphosate, and this has had massive consequences. Glyphosate is toxic to helpful gut bacteria and also breaks the bonds between gut barrier cells—which is probably why it's so effective against pests. Not shockingly, the rate of wheat allergy and celiac disease has increased in step with glyphosate use. In the past, about 1 in 133 people worldwide were estimated to suffer from these conditions. Now it's as high as 1 in 7.[20] As with any drug, the toxicity to babies is the worst, and yet most infant cereal is made from nonorganic grains.

I used to be a supporter of nonorganic farming because I thought that without these innovations, we were doomed to have periodic famines. However bad allergic diseases are, the thought of malnourished, starving children seemed worse. But it turns out that rather than preventing famine, industrial farming ensures that we will produce only soy and corn, that those foods will be turned into fillers, and that corn syrup will land in our children's bellies while leaving them starved for actual nutrition. Even worse, as we throw away about a third of the food we grow, there are still massive famines worldwide.

One of the reasons it's been so hard to prove that toxins are bad is that not everyone is equally sensitive to sugar, dyes, or pesticides. Some people can eat a hundred times the amount of glyphosate that another person can. Scientists aren't sure why this is the case. Perhaps some children's microbiomes are more disrupted than that of others, causing them to have leaky gut syndrome. Or perhaps, just as with medicine, each person can react differently to the same dose of something. What I do know is that between my two sons, one can eat anything without any problems and the other cannot at all. Because of this difference in my own house, I long thought food toxins couldn't possibly explain one son's disruptive behavior. Once I made the connection between illnesses and the microbiome, though, it seemed obvious that we should remove anything from his diet that could be harmful to the gut bacteria.

Within a day of removing preservatives, dyes, and pesticides from our house, we saw a change in Leo's behavior. Instead of having multiple tantrums a day, he had one a week or less. Everyone who knew him well remarked how much better he could regulate his emotions. It's clear that once he wasn't in constant pain, controlling his feelings was simply much easier. This good pattern continues today as long as he eats clean.

But I have such guilt about the past. I think about his critical early years, the time during which 80 percent of his brain developed, when I continually harmed him by giving him the wrong food. Each tantrum led to increased stress and fighting that I'm sure did nothing good for his brain development. He was even deprived of happy experiences because we resisted going out to do fun things. Leo's behavior out of the house—when we would eat the most packaged food—could be exhausting, and frankly, embarrassing for him and us.

We thought we ate really well, and for three out of four of us it *was* healthy. But for one of our family, it was not. Avoiding sweeteners, pesticides, dyes, and preservatives can be really difficult, especially if you are constrained by time or money. But there is no way that sugar or pesticides could possibly be good for anyone's microbiome, and each family has to choose how far to go to remove these things within their constraints.

....

What to Feed Your Child

If you can't eat processed and packaged foods, which take up most of the footprint in any grocery store, what can you eat? *New York Times* bestselling author Michael Pollan said it best with this simple explanation: "Eat food. Not too much. Mostly plants." For decades, we have known that a diet high in fiber, made up mostly of vegetables, fruits, and lean protein, is the key to good health. We now know that the reason this diet is healthy is that fibrous foods feed the commensal bacteria we have evolved with. These bacteria line our gut with protective mucus, help regulate our immune system, and communicate messages to our brain.

Studies back up the fact that our highly processed diet, so lacking in beneficial fiber, is hurting our microbiome. People in industrialized Western countries (such as the United States, Canada, and Western Europe) have gut biomes that are distinct from people in non-Western countries (in Africa and parts of South America, for example).[21] What's the result of this? Non-Westerners experience fewer autoimmune issues.

> **A diet high in fiber, made up mostly of vegetables, fruits, and lean protein, is the key to good health.**

High *Prevotella* levels are associated with diets that are high in fiber and complex carbohydrates and lower in fats and animal protein. A study of the guts of ancient humans using fossilized stools and biopsies showed that humans for most of their history have also had primarily *Prevotella* and, more frequently, multiple groups of species.

What the study also illustrated was that Westerners have fewer *Prevotella* bacteria—including a smaller number of species—and instead have *Bacteroides* bacteria in their guts. People in non-Western countries typically have two to four groups (clades) of *Prevotella* species in their guts, whereas people in Western countries have one or none. In sum, we are totally missing key bacteria that calm our immune systems.

Is there any doubt that the microbiome and the food we eat are deeply interrelated?

The vital connection between food and health is why every popular diet plan says the same thing with slight variations. Eat fewer grains, eat no refined grains, consume a mix of animal protein or plant protein and vegetables, eat some probiotic fermented foods, and never buy food with powdered cheese, preservatives, or sugar.

Many of us feel like we don't have time to cook, don't know how to prepare it, and will never, ever get our kids to eat anything that doesn't come from a box. But I want to be clear about something that you are not going to like. The only way to eat well is to cook or prepare almost all your food. That includes breakfast and lunches, not just dinners. Premade packaged meals and snacks will only cause dysbiosis of the gut.

The only way to eat well is to cook or prepare almost all your food. That includes breakfast and lunches, not just dinners.

Which diet you choose will depend on how much your family prefers meats or vegetables. I don't want to be overly prescriptive about what children should eat because no clinical study has ever proven that a specific set of recipes is the key to health. You should feel free to pick among the amazing number of cookbooks on clean eating. I will stick to practical advice to prioritize healthy brain, immune, and gut development, such as:

1. **Start at Home**
   Pediatric nutritionist Jill Castle says to "make your home a health haven." That means buying organic (when possible) fruits, vegetables, whole grains, and lean meats. Keep all snacks, sodas, and cookies out of your grocery cart and out of the house. Don't stress out too much about what happens outside the home, though. If your children eat 90 percent of their meals from a healthy home base, it's okay if they have French fries, dessert, and other foods in the remaining 10 percent of the meals they eat outside of it.

2. **Remember That Toddlers Are Not Adults**
   Toddlers do not need high levels of protein in their diet like adults, and they should have no added sugar at all for the first two years. Toddlers are also not ready for a fixed routine; they need to explore many different tastes and textures, so let them try a lot of things. Eating a variety of foods is one of the best ways to ensure that they are getting enough iron for their brains, calcium for their bones, and fiber for their guts.
   Researchers from the American Gut Project[22] found that regularly eating thirty-plus different types of plant foods per week created a more diverse microbiome than eating ten or fewer different plant foods a week. (Again, a more diverse diet means a more diverse microbiome with way more helpful species.) You may think that toddlers won't be able to handle

this many servings, but remember that a single grape and a slice of an orange count as two! Almost everyone eats twenty-one meals each week, and most toddlers hit twenty-eight to thirty-five. Adding a small amount of fruit or vegetables to each meal is a great way to ensure they are getting variety and that most of their diet consists of vegetables and fruits.

3. Stop Mindless Eating

Jill Castle states that if you are eating a protein bar for every breakfast and your child is eating animal crackers each time they are in a stroller, you should stop and ask yourself why. Mindless eating almost always includes ultra-processed foods full of sugars. We never mindlessly eat homemade curry. Toddlers are exhausting, and it can feel hard at first to be intentional about meals. But if meals become a source of joy—a fun part of each day, instead of something to get through—then it's easier. I myself am an "eat to live" rather than a "live to eat" sort of person, but making time for a sit-down meal actually provides families with a great way to connect.

A friend told me recently that her family (with two young children) plays a little game when they sit down to dinner. Each person gets the chance to list the "rose" and the "thorn" of their day. Recounting their highs and lows not only makes each of them feel special and listened to but also buys a few minutes when their kids are guaranteed to focus and not pick at their food or complain.

4. Train for Adulthood

Babies and toddlers need different nutrients than adults do, but they are in training to eat as adults. That means that meals should be at a table, with family, as often as possible. The whole family should eat the same thing, even if your toddler eats only some of it and in small quantities. When you are an adult, no one forces you to eat anything, and similarly, toddlers should be offered a plate of healthy food, but not made to finish a plate when they are full or unhappy with flavors they haven't grown used to. It's fine to insist they try, but don't push them to finish a plate, because it will only cause more heartache than good.

The idea of training your baby to eat like an adult may be the most critical component of healthy eating. A generation ago, parents used to spank their children. We now understand that if we want children to grow up with respect for others and avoid violence, we need to lead by example and not inflict violence on them. Eating is the same. If we want to raise adults that enjoy food and respect their own hunger and nutrition cues, we cannot force-feed them or turn meals into stressful battles.

Do not feed your child "kid food" like nuggets and mac 'n' cheese. These foods won't be their favorites if they never have them. Rather, offer them the same flavorful, healthy items on your plate. Get them to think of flavors—even spices—as a normal part of good food. Give them agency by letting them decide what goes in today's rice bowl, burritos, or casserole. And as they go through phases where they want to eat more or less, or try new things or not, be patient. Remember that healthy eating, like any other adult habit, takes years of encouragement and reinforcement. Sometime between eighteen and thirty-six months is when the gut microbiome shifts to a more stable profile that sets a child up for a lifetime of obesity and other chronic disease—or not.[23] Choose wisely.

> Do not feed your child "kid food" like nuggets and mac 'n' cheese. These foods won't be their favorites if they never have them.

....

Do Probiotics Work?

Probiotics are refined, concentrated microbes, and their active ingredient is often combined with helper chemicals. They come in pill, powder, and liquid form, and how effective they are depends on whether you get a well-made product with useful strains, what percentage of the microbes actually make it into your system, and how your diet and lifestyle choices either assist or limit the product's effectiveness.

While it's helpful to think of probiotics as you would any other medicine or drug, there are some limitations to the probiotic industry. I don't want to say that probiotics today are the snake oil of the pharmaceutical industry, but that's probably not a terrible analogy, either. There are definitely companies out there making great products, but a lot of what's on the shelves is garbage. Unlike drugs, however, "bad" probiotics seem to be relatively harmless.

It's not all bad news, though. Thanks to our exploding understanding of the microbiome, the probiotic industry is rapidly evolving. Scientists are working on better products backed by real clinical studies of their efficacy and have regulated manufacturing standards. As was true in the 1800s—when we were first developing respect for drugs and their benefits—today we are realizing that the best drug for many conditions may actually be a bacterium. Several companies are developing medical-grade probiotics with strains they have isolated and proven to prevent or reverse diseases. In the skin care area, companies are moving from salicylic acid to destroy skin bacteria to probiotic serums of macrophages that discretely eat *Cutibacterium acnes*.

These are just two examples in the larger, rapidly shifting field of microbe-based medicine. It's crazy to think that ten years ago, probiotics were a punch-line poop joke about fecal transplants. Today, large clinical studies are being done and microbe drugs are a full-fledged part of the biotech industry. That pipeline is full of promise and excitement about the prospect that we can prevent, treat, and cure immune disease.

Until then, parents should approach the probiotic aisle of the grocery store with a healthy mix of hope and skepticism. And when you go shopping, you need to ask four things:

1. Are you hoping the probiotic is like a drug that will fix something or more like a vitamin to better your health?
2. Is there scientific proof that the strains in the probiotic will do what you want? The wrong bacterial strain is as useless as taking a cholesterol drug for healthy skin.
3. Does the probiotic have the right combination of dose, or colony-forming units (CFUs), and other ingredients to better your health? What other ingredients does it contain, and will these be harmful to you?
4. Could diet (or sleep, exercise, or time) be as effective as taking a probiotic?

Let's start with the goal of treatment versus health, and what a probiotic can and can't do for both. Because research on probiotics is in its infancy, most of the broad-spectrum probiotics available today can't treat the problems you already have. Instead, they are best used like vitamins to support ongoing health.

Why? Because when you add a particular bacterium to your system, it can't implant itself in your gut lining if the gut is already occupied by other bacteria. In many clinical studies of probiotics, researchers start by having participants take a large dose of antibiotics to kill off existing bacteria and create space for the microbe in the study. In functional medicine, a provider will often ask their patient to simultaneously take a probiotic and an extract that is intended to kill off other bacteria or fungi. Or they may ask their patient to change their diet to starve unwanted species.

Naturopathic physician Dr. Carrie Runde says that for chronic health concerns, she rarely uses probiotics instead of diet or lifestyle changes. As she puts it, these "are different tools with different long-term effects and can be used together if indicated. Lifestyle changes are the most foundational for chronic health issues like allergies, digestive concerns, and skin complaints. For example, children with constipation are often impacted by low water and fiber intake, combined with fear around stooling due to a history of painful bowel movements. So we work on these issues first. Additionally, overexposure to oral prescription antibiotics, food sensitivities, and excessive sugar consumption are common factors for children with digestive problems. A probiotic may help with constipation, depending on the exact strain, but is not going to fix diet and lifestyle issues for most kids."

When most people go shopping for probiotics, they aren't working with a provider to do something to create space for the probiotic species, so the probiotics won't be as helpful as a treatment. There are some exceptions to this, however. Many people successfully use broad-spectrum gut probiotics after a course of antibiotics to reset their guts. Dr. Runde adds, "A probiotic is going to have an impact on health for the duration of consumption, plus a week after stopping it. There are situations where use of a probiotic is the best route because of the self-limited nature of the health issue. A great example of this is the use of probiotics while a kid is on a course of prescription antibiotics. Giving researched strains of probiotics concurrently, but not in the same swallow as the antibiotic, can prevent gastrointestinal side effects."

In infants, whose guts are rapidly changing and looking for new species, the right probiotics can also be useful. But even then, they act more like vitamins to prevent future problems instead of reversing existing ones.

The second reason to avoid most probiotics is that manufacturers can legally sell only GRAS (generally regarded as safe) bacteria that are already found in food. Many brands also sell only probiotics with species-level controls. When it comes to bacteria, it's not the species that matter to your health but the strains. Imagine calling for help with an electrical problem and hearing, "Sure, we'll send a human, but we can't guarantee they have any electrical training!" Only a couple of strains of bacteria available today have clinical data showing they can fix or prevent things like allergic disease,[24] and only certain strains of *Lactobacillus rhamnosus* have been shown to reduce the risk of eczema.[25]

You should always check the bottle to find out what strains are being used and whether those strains have clinical data to show that they are effective. As Dr. Runde puts it: "The most important factor when picking a probiotic is to find an organism and strain that are researched for your specific health concern (constipation, gas, seasonal allergies, etc.). If the label does not specify the strain of probiotic and just lists the genus and species, that is a warning sign that they're not using a researched strain in their probiotic. It should be listed on the label (i.e., *Lactobacillus rhamnosus* HN001) under the nutrition facts."

Check a probiotic to find out what strains are being used and whether those strains have clinical data to show that they are effective.

You should also check to be sure a probiotic is appropriate for the person's age. Some strains of *Lactobacillus rhamnosus, Bifidobacterium breve, B. lactis,* and *B. infantis* are relevant for babies' developing systems, while other strains of bacteria may only be helpful for adults.

The third concern is content. As mentioned earlier, most probiotics have not been found to be harmful—other than wasting your money. It may not hurt that a brand has 2 billion CFUs of this and 1 billion CFUs of that, but it also may not help. Some strains can need as many as 15 billion CFUs per day to have an effect.

On the other hand, more CFUs aren't necessarily better. Some brands will advertise 20 billion CFU, but it might be spread across several strains, which doesn't help. Not all bacteria play nice with one another, so jamming in many strains may not be as useful as combining a probiotic with prebiotic food for the bacteria.

The last thing to consider about contents is that most probiotics, like drugs, have to have other ingredients to be shelf stable. Infant probiotics, usually given as liquid drops, need a carrier liquid that can vary from pure organic sunflower oil to less desirable chemicals.

Finally, the fourth consideration to make about commercially available probiotics today also applies to medicine. We know Advil can reduce pain, but so can rest and ice. And Advil won't really help if you keep hurting yourself again and again. Prevention can be the best medicine.

It's important to remember that any probiotic use must be supported by the diet choices discussed in this chapter. Throwing fresh paint on your wall will not do much if you are continually taking a wrecking ball to that same wall with artificial sweeteners and pesticides. And given that most probiotics only give you strains that grow in food, today you may be better off regularly adding probiotic foods, rather than supplements, to your diet. Every culture has their version—yogurt, kefir, kombucha, kimchi, pickles, sauerkraut, and more—so you can find one with a flavor profile, texture, and fermentation process that works in your house. Remember that commensal bacteria live on fiber from fruits and vegetables and that they require the amino acids in animal proteins and beans to thrive. Probiotic foods mean that you are eating live, healthy, commensal bacteria made from ingredients that facilitate their growth instead of freeze-dried bacteria. In essence, you are eating their food as you eat the bacteria itself.

....

In Conclusion

We all know that we are what we eat. A healthy diet that supports a strong immune-regulating microbiome is one very low in sugar and made of real food, including vegetables, fruits, animal or plant protein, and whole grains. This is the diet that humans have had for millennia, varied only by which animal proteins and plants were locally available. Modern food preservation using chemicals didn't exist until recently, and no one's microbiome has caught up to tolerate it. Our commensal bacteria may evolve to love glyphosate one day, but you and I do not have the luxury of waiting. Our children most especially don't have it.

A clean diet does not have to be more expensive than an unhealthy diet. Implying that good foods are for the privileged is a false narrative that has been peddled to keep people eating corn byproducts. Fruits and vegetables in season are cheaper per pound than packaged foods, as are grains and dried beans in bulk. Homemade spice mixes are cheaper than "flavor packets." Moreover, money spent on immune disease prevention is significantly less expensive than the doctors, ER visits, medications, and specialists required to manage disease for the rest of your child's life. I have the medical receipts to prove it.

If you have gotten this far and believe that the microbiome is important to preventing a whole category of diseases, then the only logical action is to minimize things that could harm the microbiome (as always, while maintaining your sanity) by investing in yourself—and most of all, investing in your child's future.

CHAPTER SIX

The Impact of the Environment

Common Misconception:
Don't let your kids play in the dirt.

A huge source of gut biome disruption is the lack of dirt in your day-to-day life. Healthy soil is your microbiome's friend because it is chock-full of helpful bacteria. Each cubic centimeter of dirt has about the same number of microbes as the equivalent volume of your intestines. A living environment without dirt will naturally leave you in less contact with microbes to "refresh" your system.

Families that live on farms are shown to have fewer allergic and autoimmune diseases. Amish communities that perform manual farming and live in close contact with animals have significantly less allergic disease than those who use machines to farm and don't live near animals.

Until I was faced with a child suffering from a mountain of diseases that had spun out of my control, I had succeeded at almost everything I had tried in my life. I had gotten into, enrolled in, and graduated from a good college. I had started and sold an orthopedic company. I had taken up triathlons and found my way to the podium. I had also been a good wife, sister, and daughter. I was never the best at anything, but I was never even *close* to the worst.

Yet here I was, trying my hardest to be a "good" mom—something I was convinced billions of other women had pulled off—and I was failing miserably because I couldn't keep my son healthy. By the time Leo was three, I could mostly control his food allergies, but being constantly vigilant was taxing. I knew all my efforts to keep him away from his triggers were destined to fail sometimes, so I lived in constant fear. Leo's eczema was generally better, but it still sometimes flared. His congestion and asthma also came and went randomly, and I was frustrated I couldn't find a pattern. Almost daily, my fruitless efforts reminded me that not everything could be in my control, and I hated that feeling.

I soon realized that there is no such thing as the perfect mom. Being a "good" mom is more about listening, being present, and showing love despite how hard things get. A child's health (or lack thereof) often has zero correlation with how "good" a parent you are. But it's frustrating to feel like a failure. I get it. And for type A people like me, a lack of control is one of the worst parts of immune diseases. While we can change our diets, say no to antibiotics, and wash our babies less often, much of what causes the dysbiosis that leads to them are environmental factors that are completely out of our hands.

Here is a case in point. A 2018 study[1] compared the gut microbiomes and health of Hmong people (an ethnic group) who resided in Thailand with Hmong people who had recently emigrated to the United States. The results proved that gut microbiomes are incredibly sensitive to where people live. The immigrants' gut microbiomes had started to shift from one that was high in *Prevotella* to one high in *Bacteroides*—a typically American biome—*within two weeks* of their arrival in the United States. The longer they stayed here, the more their guts looked like American guts. In addition, the first generation of children of Hmong immigrants born in the United States had gut microbiomes that were effectively the same as those of children whose families had been here for generations.

What's strangest about this shift from *Prevotella* to *Bacteroides* is that it happened no matter what the immigrants ate. *Even if immigrants continued eating the foods from their country of origin, their microbiome changed.* In fact, researchers concluded that only about 16 percent of the alteration of their microbial population could be attributed to diet alone.

Clearly, something else out there was changing the microbiome, and undoubtedly the epithelial barriers, of the Hmong people, but we don't know what. Research bears out the fact that the external, environmental influences on a child—especially from toddlerhood on—are as important as the personal and dietary ones on their risk of immune disease. The environment children grow up in is a significant driver of their microbiome and epithelial barrier integrity, especially after they have settled into an adult diet. All the interventions I've discussed so far matter greatly and add up as part of the big picture, but we must add the environment—including water, air, the outside, and the home—to the story.

The previous three chapters—on antibiotics, baby care practices in the first six months, and diet—have given you ways that you can *directly* reduce the risk of dysbiosis and barrier dysfunction.

....

External, environmental influences on a child—especially from toddlerhood on—are as important as the personal and dietary ones on their risk of immune disease.

....

This chapter is much less empowering in that so many of the issues it discusses are not in our immediate control. However, by taking steps at the local level and in your home, you can feel confident that in your own small way, you can still work toward a healthier world for you and your children.

....

How to Ensure Your Water Is Safe

While babies typically aren't given plain water in their bottles, water is used to make formula. After a baby has been weaned, water is the only fluid children (and adults) should regularly drink.

Since the Safe Drinking Water Act was enacted in 1974, the Environmental Protection Agency (EPA) has actively worked to ensure that drinking water is safe and free from naturally occurring and man-made contaminants. Because of this law and its enforcement, water is probably the least likely source of environmentally caused dysbiosis. It is also the environmental concern easiest to fix—if that's what's needed.

But real problems do occur with water. All of the chemicals or microparticles in your water may be harmful to your microbiome, or they may be damaging the "mortar" between your barrier cells directly.

Cities with aging pipes or lead-lined pipes can end up with contaminated water. Rainwater from fields, lawns, and work sites drains into local waterways, as does chemical runoff from health care facilities and production facilities. While treatment plants are designed to remove most of the offending chemicals, many streams, wells, and municipal water systems that are tested showed levels of pesticides above the EPA's allowable threshold.[2]

Even with these findings, know that your tap water is probably fine. The Environmental Working Group (EWG), a nonprofit environmental advocacy organization, suggests that Americans should drink tap water unless there is an environmental disaster that overwhelms the water management system (like a hurricane) or a water crisis (like the lead contamination crisis that occurred in Flint, Michigan, from 2014 to 2019).

> **The Environmental Working Group suggests that Americans should drink tap water unless there is an environmental disaster.**

Nonetheless, water quality varies from city to city and state to state, and some areas score higher than others in terms of the number of pollutants that are in their municipal water. What can you do about this? First, you can read the research on water quality that arrives in your mailbox. According to the EPA, almost all community water systems mail out an annual Consumer Confidence Report each July. This report outlines all pollutants and contaminants in your local water, along with their possible health effects. If you do not receive something, the EPA encourages you to call your local water supplier. Many of these suppliers also offer free water testing (with kits provided!) or you can Google epa.gov for the EPA's latest guidance on the safety of ground and drinking water in your area. Lastly, you can call the Safe Drinking Water Hotline at 1-800-426-4791.

Regardless of how much research or testing you do on your own, know that the water you drink should contain trace minerals and few to no pathogens. Filtered tap water is significantly healthier than bottled water, which has spent excessive time in plastic that can leach chemicals into it. If you want to further reduce any possible toxic effect to gut bacteria from ingested chemicals or heavy metals, it's a good idea to invest in a filter. Information contained on the Environmental Working Group's database[3] on water systems, as well as your local Consumer Confidence Report, will help you know what kind of—if any—filter to purchase.

Carbon filters, including countertop pitcher filters and refrigerator filters, work by binding chemicals in the water to the carbon in the filter. Some carbon filters only reduce chlorine and improve taste and odor, while others can decrease levels of asbestos, lead, mercury, and volatile organic compounds (VOCs). Carbon filters are typically inexpensive, but you should note that they do not remove inorganic pollutants such as arsenic, fluoride, hexavalent chromium, nitrate, and perchlorate.

Reverse osmosis filters—which you install in your house to filter all your water pipes—are significantly more expensive. They use a two-step process to remove chlorine, trihalomethanes, and VOCs, as well as any particles larger than water molecules. Reverse osmosis effectively removes inorganic pollutants carbon filters cannot, but it also pulls out trace minerals that you *do* want in your water. Reverse osmosis systems are also incredibly wasteful because they flush out four times the water than gets used.

Finally, most tap water contains added fluoride to help reduce tooth decay. Fluoride is a natural mineral and is found in most toothpastes and mouthwashes. Very large doses of fluoride can cause side effects, such as white spots on the teeth and skeletal fluorosis, but to date no studies have shown a link between fluoride and allergic or autoimmune disease. One study showed that even at fluoride levels 2.5 times the norm, no adverse health effects were seen.[4]

....

The Importance of Dirt

Scott and I have lived in the same house, in a neighborhood that was once home to a number of factories, since Leo was born. When he was a baby, we didn't know what kind of toxic waste might be lurking in the soil, so we were nervous about letting him get into the dirt in our backyard. Then we had the soil tested by the University of Delaware Soil Testing Program, saw that it was fine, and felt comfortable letting him crawl around.

We do live in a city, though, so what we call our backyard would be simply a patch of grass to most people. Plus, cities aren't exactly known for their abundance of natural terrain. When Leo was ready to run around, we spent a lot of time at city playgrounds with artificial surfaces instead of grass, play sets instead of trees, and splash pads instead of creeks. In theory, we could have driven to greener spaces or spent more time in public parks, but it often didn't work between naps or with our schedules. Besides, play spaces felt better designed for a toddler who was already prone to getting messy.

I'll never know for sure if my choice to go to the playground rather than the park contributed to Leo's immune diseases, but it didn't help. Leo had access to good dirt but probably didn't get enough of it, and if I had to do it all over, I'd take him to real parks as much as I could.

A lack of dirt in your day-to-day life is an important source of environmentally caused dysbiosis. Healthy soil is your microbiome's friend because it is chock-full of the same commensal bacteria that allow your body to thrive. Each cubic centimeter of dirt has about the same number of microbes as the equivalent volume of your intestines,[5] so it goes to figure that an environment without dirt naturally leaves you in less contact with microbes to "refresh" your system.[6] Without those microbes, your barriers break down, allowing immune diseases to flourish.

Healthy soil is your microbiome's friend because it is chock-full of the same commensal bacteria that allow your body to thrive.

Studies bear this out, and families that live on farms are shown to have fewer allergic and autoimmune diseases.[7] Amish communities who perform manual farming and live in close contact with animals have significantly less allergic disease than the otherwise similar Hutterite communities, who live in Montana, North and South Dakota, Minnesota, and western Canada. Why the difference in the rate of allergic disease? The Hutterites use machines to farm, so they interact less with the dirt, and they don't live near animals, who are covered in it.[8]

A similar difference can be seen in the general population. Children growing up in urban settings are three to five times more likely to end up in the ER from anaphylaxis than children growing up in rural areas,[9] where children spend more time in dirt. The problem isn't exclusive to humans, either; domesticated animals like horses and creatures living in zoos also show less gut diversity than their wild counterparts.[10]

For most of history, humans have lived in close contact with dirt either because they were farmers or simply because it was inescapable, so no one thought much about what is actually *in* dirt. As we grew aware of microbial pathogens, toxic waste, and—for those of you who grew up in the 1980s—the dreaded hypodermic needles that were rumored to litter the soil of urban areas, we began limiting the amount of dirt children were exposed to.

We must remember that many of our commensal bacteria are also potential pathogens. As I mentioned in chapter 2, the presence of *Escherichia coli*—a bacterium whose side effects range from diarrhea to death—also protects Russian Karelian children from immune malfunction. Their systems don't take in the *E. coli* from breast milk, and they don't receive it from food contamination, since that would cause them to get sick. Most likely, these Russian children get small amounts of *E. coli* through their exposure to dirt. After all, Karelian society is rooted in forestry, outdoor activities, and the land.

If you have access to good soil, by which I mean natural parks with trees and clean streams, let your child play in it. Let them touch the microbes in the dirt and get them on their skin. Encourage your kids to dig in mud, roll in grass, and splash in streams. Let your children garden with you, and swap out the sand in your covered sandbox for dirt free of pesticides and chemicals. Your kid will love getting messy, and while you may dread cleaning out the tub after bath time, you can rest easy knowing that your child got some good exposure to bacteria. All these activities have been shown to be associated with lower rates of allergic and autoimmune disease.[11] Simply spending time outside also has been demonstrated to have positive effects on emotional regulation and focus.

It's important to put the benefit of dirt into context. Dirt full of chemicals like lead and pesticides is worse for your child's health than no dirt. If your home or town has been continuously populated for a hundred years, the dirt in your backyard is likely quite clean. However, if you douse your lawn in pesticides and fertilizer four times a year, it is no longer safe. Dirt with chemicals in it contains different microbes than dirt without pesticides. Furthermore, if your property is newer, check to see how that land was used before assuming the dirt is clean. Many newer neighborhoods are built on former industrial sites or landfills, meaning the dirt can be low quality and even polluted.

If dirt is so good, then why did I spend a bunch of time convincing you to wash your hands to avoid unnecessary infections?

To be clear, infants in Russian Karelia do not get harmful *E. coli* infections when they play in the dirt. In dirt, *E. coli* is a commensal bacterium that helps the gut. But these same children—and your children, too—can very likely pick up pathogenic viruses from touching public bathrooms and day care toys, which are crawling with them.

Finally, if dirt is so good, why am I still living in the middle of a city? It would be easy to suggest that we simply leave our home and move to a house with a bigger yard, but life is never without trade-offs. The towns we might be able to afford create a commute of an hour and a half both ways, meaning that we would be far more sedentary and certainly more exhausted every day. And there's no guarantee that the dirt in a suburb is necessarily clean; many Philadelphia suburbs have tested positive for chemical runoff from industrial plants and even nuclear energy sites. Many people living in urban areas face a similar dilemma or simply don't have access to a state park or forest. If you can't travel, then remember that limiting exposure to things that harm the microbiome is important and that you can continuously support the microbiome through a good diet, including probiotic foods. As with everything, do the best you can for your child. Go to the local park. Play in the dirt. Soak up the sunshine and know you've done your research, weighed the pros and cons of your choices, and picked your battles. If you've done that, you are absolutely helping your child live a healthy, happy life.

....

The Home Environment

Since most of us spend the majority of our days inside, our home environment plays a big role in shaping our microbiome.[12]

The microbes in the home come from the people and animals

who bring it in from the outdoors. This can be a bad thing. My parents were raised in India, where if you weren't diligent about cleaning floors and taking your shoes off when you entered your home, you were asking for filth. They raised me and my sister with the same philosophy, and in our house, we mopped floors each night and vacuumed every crevice on the weekends. I'm sure this was overkill, but today Scott and I maintain a "no shoes in the house" policy because data shows that's a smart move in a city. In Philadelphia, wearing shoes in the home is a leading cause of lead poisoning in infants. In other towns, that might be less of a concern, so do your research.

A study in Germany showed that fungus brought in from the outdoors is associated with the development of behavioral problems during childhood. Poorly cleaned homes often had a diverse fungal environment living on the floors, counters, carpets, and walls, and this increased the likelihood of ADHD.[13] If you have any mold or fungus in your house, address this right away. Mold and fungus can cause many illnesses well beyond immune conditions. And bear in mind if you have water damage in your home—whether from a leaking pipe, an upstairs neighbor who let the tub overflow, or a flood—be sure to get the walls and ceiling tested for mold growth. Just because you can't see mold or fungus doesn't mean it's not blossoming in a cold, wet, hidden area.

I now know that Leo has definitely had some kind of sensitivity to mold from the time he was five. We first thought he was developing seasonal allergies because he always seemed congested in the spring. But the congestion would last into the summer. We tested him several times for pollen allergies, but they all came up negative.

Recently, after keeping a journal, I noticed that Leo's congestion and skin flares were worst when it rained or was excessively humid. It rains a lot in the spring, and the summers in

Philadelphia can be exceedingly humid. Of course mold and fungus thrive in these conditions. I connected the dots and realized that if Leo wasn't allergic to whatever bloomed in the spring and summer, it had to be something else. Scott and I ordered mold tests in our home, and sure enough, we had mold we couldn't see or smell. We dealt with it, and Leo's eczema and congestion improved.

While the German study I mentioned earlier in this chapter pointed out how harmful fungal growth can be, it also bore out the fact that the microbes in our homes can be beneficial. Researchers swabbed the floors of their subjects' houses and discovered that the diverse colonies of bacteria on them had a direct correlation with a lower incidence of ADHD. The microbes that are on your floor populate your child's gut and allow the richness of the microbiome to replenish itself. Children who live in families with dogs who go outside also have more diverse microbiomes[14] and fewer immune diseases than those who don't because animals track dirt into the house from outside. Having other pets (like fish or gerbils) that stay inside makes no difference. Finally, children who grow up with siblings—meaning there's at least twice as much kid-tracked dirt in the house—are also less likely to develop allergic diseases.[15]

How we choose to clean our homes, dishes, and clothes may be the biggest cause of immune disorders. The ingredients in laundry detergent, dishwashing detergent, and bathroom/kitchen cleaning products have been shown to be directly toxic to our epithelial barriers, not just the microbiome that supports them. Two recent studies looked at the damage to barrier cells of the skin and lungs from laundry detergents.[16] Even when the detergents were diluted, meaning a teensy bit was placed in a huge amount of water, the detergents caused changes to the cells and invoked immune responses.

The two biggest culprit chemicals are sodium dodecyl sulfate and sodium dodecylbenzene sulfonate, which damage the barriers of the skin and lungs even in trace amounts. These compounds are found in many soaps, shampoos, detergents, and cleaning agents. Both are easily found on towels and clothes after washing or use, meaning you are being constantly exposed to them.

> **How we choose to clean our homes, dishes, and clothes may be the biggest cause of immune disorders.**

After I learned about these harmful ingredients, we switched from conventional detergent to oxygen bleach, a laundry soap that contains only sodium carbonate and sodium citrate and is basically just baking soda. We wipe counters with plain water and maybe vinegar, and we use only natural soap and shampoos. This switch was frustrating at times; it took me years to find a shampoo and conditioner that didn't make me look like a wet dog, for example. I've also struggled to find the right dishwasher detergent, so I've settled on an easy fix: washing dishes by hand and using the dishwasher as more of a drying space.

Antibacterial Cleansers and Public Health

When I was writing this book, my family and I decided to take a spring break trip to Disney World. It was March 2021, and we were one year into the COVID-19 pandemic. My husband and I weren't yet vaccinated—the vaccine rollout for thirty-somethings with no comorbidities didn't start in earnest in Pennsylvania until April 2021—but we felt that the chance of any of us catching the virus while walking outside, wearing masks, in a mostly uncrowded park was small.

Disney theme parks are famously well run and maintained,

but I was still shocked at how sparkling clean the place was when we got there. There were gloved, masked employees everywhere scooping up trash and wiping railings. There were hand-sanitizing stations everywhere, and you were required to use them before boarding a ride. Park employees scrubbed down every ride every hour with disinfecting wipes and spray. The bathrooms smelled like bleach, and you weren't allowed to get within six feet of Mickey, Minnie, or any character wandering the park.

For five straight days, we rode all the rides we could and had a blast, and we didn't get sick, just as we'd expected. But while immersing ourselves in that unnaturally sterile environment, coating ourselves with hand sanitizer every half hour, what harm did we inflict on our microbiomes?

Unfortunately, during the COVID-19 pandemic, *safe* became conflated with "you should scrub all surfaces and your hands with toxic chemicals that wipe out every helpful pathogen that lives on them." For the first time since 1904 (and at an annual cost of $300 million), the New York City subway closed for four hours every night so employees could disinfect train cars and stations from top to bottom. Officials even bragged they used germ-killing ultraviolet light. To make airplane travel "safe," airlines sanitized every plane after every trip with harsh chemicals and electrostatic technology. Even though scientists and the CDC made it clear that the virus is airborne and that the chance of catching it via surface transmission is only one out of ten thousand, grocery stores ran out of disinfecting wipes daily, and everyone began using hand sanitizer like it was going out of style.

While the world we live in became shiny, clean, and germ-free in 2020, scientists now agree it happened at the expense of our biomes. A January 2021 paper published in the *Proceedings of the National Academy of Science of the USA* warned that over-cleaning, physical separation, and travel restrictions may have wiped out entire populations of microbes and severely restricted the ability of others to colonize.[17] While the effects of this microbial loss is still unknown, scientists fear that the health of the general population will suffer in the long term.

The only way to reverse this dangerous trend, scientists warn, is to work as hard as possible to go back to the hygiene practices we had before the pandemic—and even improve on them. We shouldn't be using hand sanitizer every five minutes, nor should we be using antibacterial wipes on every doorknob in our homes once a day. We can return to shaking hands as long as we remember to wash them with soap and water before we eat. And we can allow our children to swing from the monkey bars, spin in the teacups at Disney, and play in the sandbox as long as they don't touch their faces and, again, always wash their hands.

....

The Air You Breathe

The one battle that we should all be picking—yet have the least ability to affect—is the battle against air pollution. While most people would never make the connection, air pollution is well documented as a leading driver of chronic and immune disease. It is the world's fourth leading cause of death, causing at least thirteen deaths a minute. Its risks have grown so blatantly clear that in September 2021, the World Health Organization revised its global air quality guidelines by cutting the recommended yearly limit of particulate matter or droplets in the air that are two and one half microns or less in width (like particles from cars, trucks, planes, and wildfire smoke) in half. Cars produce a complex mixture of air pollutants including carbon monoxide, nitrogen oxides, particulate matter, volatile organic compounds (like benzene), and other hazardous air pollutants (HAPs).[18] At least thirteen studies have shown that the quantity of these chemicals that children breathe is directly related to their risk of asthma, eczema, and hay fever.[19] Air pollution has even been shown to cause infertility.[20]

Air pollution is well documented as a leading driver of chronic and immune disease.

We are not totally sure how air pollution causes immune disease.[21] It is possible that these chemicals are toxic to the bacteria on your skin and in your airways, changing how your body responds to non-harmful substances. It is also possible that the chemicals directly trigger our immune cells, causing them to overreact.[22] Other studies have suggested that fine particulates and ozone cause mutations in the barrier cells similar to the way that air pollution can lead to cancer.

Though the Clean Air Act of 1963 was supposed to prevent Americans from having to deal with the known and unknown effects of air pollution, particulates in the air are significantly harder to manage than water contamination. Exposure to traffic-related chemicals can happen if you live near a major roadway or if you spend an excessive amount of time in a car.[23] Pollution from cars affects both those of us who live in cities near highways or big roads and those of us who live far from cities and end up driving more. Air pollution can blow from industrial facilities far away and even come from natural sources like forest fires, thereby affecting us no matter where we live.

No matter how it gets to you, your lungs and immune system were not designed to handle air pollution. And there's almost nothing you can do about it. Very few of us can financially or practically afford a lifestyle where we are both surrounded by trees and able to avoid driving. Plus, those of us who are least able to afford the ill effects of air pollution are also probably the ones most likely to be dealing with it.

The best thing you can do is plant trees in your neighborhood, especially to line large roadways and parks. Trees are nature's natural air filters, and they also increase oxygen levels, which can change the makeup of the microbes in your environment.

Just be careful to plant trees that are native to your part of the world and to plant *both male and female trees*. Back in the 1950s, the USDA *Yearbook of Agriculture* suggested that "for street plantings, only male trees should be selected, to avoid the nuisance from the seed." Male-only trees, shrubs, and even houseplant clones were bred to satisfy demand. The problem is that male trees produce abundant allergenic pollen, and there are no female trees to capture the pollen and remove it from the air we breathe. While trees do clean the air, they can also spit those toxins back out into the air through their pollen. School yards and lawns are sometimes the most allergenic[24] places in a neighborhood, with pollen counts off the charts. We may not enjoy the sticky fruit that falls to the ground from trees, but planting a natural balance of trees will clean your air while protecting your immune system.

....

Change the System

The interventions discussed in this book thus far are decisions and actions parents themselves can implement to protect their children. But the environment is obviously bigger than any individual. Even in the food wonderland of Europe, where harmful chemicals and ingredients are banned from food, allergic and autoimmune diseases are on the rise, likely due in part to air pollution. To combat chronic disease, we *all* need to make a shift not only in our thinking but in our environments.

In the United States, across industries, we have to adopt the

precautionary principle of assuming new chemicals are dangerous unless proven otherwise. All studies of safety should look at
effects on the immune system as an early indicator of probable
disease in the future. Even chemicals, compounds, and plastics
that we currently consider to be safe should be reevaluated for
their potential to trigger immune responses. Businesses should
use only chemicals we know to be safe, and even then should be
required to filter them out of water rather than simply dumping
them into the water system for municipalities to clean up. In
Flint, for example, we have seen how aging infrastructure is
sometimes not up to the task, whereas brand-new industrial
facilities can have the capabilities built in.

A way to achieve this shift in mindset is to think about the
chemicals in our surroundings as possible immunogens, the
same way we started to question which chemicals were carcinogens. Industries today are held liable for polluting our environments with carcinogens, and the same system can help remove
immunogens from our environments.

But parents must advocate for this kind of change. Write your
members of Congress and state representatives. Vote for environmentally friendly candidates. If you have money to give,
donate it to organizations that help protect our children's immune systems.

On the flip side of removing immune triggers from our environments, we can actively work to *create* better surroundings
that provide what our bodies and microbiomes need to be
healthy. Many cities have realized that green space improves the
environment, creates biodiversity, reduces air pollution, ensures
water storage, dampens noise, and helps keep areas cool in summer heat. Almost every city in the United States is regreening,
planting more trees, converting lots into parks, and reserving
acres of land for public use as parks.

Improving the environment also reduces the enormous financial burden of treating and managing immune and other chronic diseases. An international team of researchers found that access to open, undeveloped land with natural vegetation or urban parks and street greenery was associated with reductions in the risk of type 2 diabetes, cardiovascular disease, premature death, and preterm birth.[25] A better environment is a win for everyone.

Every child should have access to clean water and outdoor spaces. Children in Flint are no more deserving of lead poisoning or immune disease than my sons, and children who live in the middle of cities need room to play in clean, safe parks just as much as those who live in the suburbs. Every child should be able to breathe clean air, too. While many of us can add filtration systems in our home, we shouldn't have to. Only after we understand that the water, dirt, and air directly affect our microbiome—and thus directly impact our health—will we truly be able to achieve real and sustained reduction in the rate of immune disease.

Public outcry did clean our waterways, remove asbestos from our living spaces, and strip lead from our gasoline, paint, and pipes. It is possible to change things that sometimes feel too big to change. Armed with this primer on the microbiome and our current epidemic of disease, I hope you will strive to protect not only your child but the children around you and the children to come.

CHAPTER SEVEN

Nurturing Your Baby's Biome During Pregnancy

> **Common Misconception:**
> If you have acid reflux during pregnancy,
> definitely take Prilosec or Nexium.
> ....

Many pregnant women experience acid reflux, which manifests as a burning in the chest when acid from the stomach bubbles up into the esophagus. Reflux is usually treated with proton pump inhibitors (PPIs) like Prilosec, Nexium, and Prevacid, all of which reduce stomach acid.

Unfortunately, PPIs may prevent proper digestion of proteins, disrupt the lining or barrier of the intestines, and change the composition of your microbiome. A series of studies in the last fifteen years have shown that acid suppression drugs taken during pregnancy are linked to an increase in childhood food allergy, food hypersensitivity, and asthma. If you are pregnant, try changing your diet or lying in an elevated position instead. Use drugs if your condition is severe, but try other methods first.

I was shocked when I found out I was pregnant with Leo. Scott and I knew we wanted to have children, and because it seemed like everyone I knew was struggling to conceive, we assumed it would be hard for us, too. So when I was thirty, we "benched the goalie," and I went off the birth control that had stopped me from menstruating (and from getting pregnant) since I was in my late teens.

"Let's see how it goes," I said to Scott. "I'm sure this won't be easy."

Wrong. I was pregnant that month. In fact, it happened so quickly that when my doctor asked, "When was your last period?" I had to honestly answer, "Twelve years ago."

When my middle got suspiciously big, I told my boss and coworkers I was pregnant. Almost immediately, it felt like I went from being the go-to problem solver to a delicate flower. I was running clinical affairs (and marketing . . . and sales . . .) at the orthopedic company I'd helped start up. I was in multiple states every week, with days that started early in surgery and ended late at steak dinners. Most weekends you could find me on my feet for hours at conferences talking to customers or with surgeons at surgical training courses, where I helped them understand the orthopedic advancements my company had developed.

Suddenly, when I became pregnant, no one let me lift anything or stand in during surgeries. My managers suggested I cut back travel and hand over conferences to others. Coming from my 100 percent male colleagues, this felt really patronizing. (Though I know in their hearts they were just trying to help.) I was also pissed off because I was still *me*, not some baby factory! I fought them and insisted on continuing to do everything I did before I was pregnant. I worked late, never called in sick, and continued to travel just as I always had. At home, I kept up my exercise routine, signed up for (and ran!) a half-marathon, repainted our entire house, and made the baby room look perfect.

While believing so fervently I was *me*, a singular human being who just happened to be carrying a fetus, I didn't fully understand just how interconnected my immune system was with my son's. Nor did I understand that while continuing to live my life and do the things I always had, I unwittingly ignored things that might have nurtured Leo's delicate developing immune system. Pregnancy does not turn you into a delicate flower, but it does change how things affect your body.

As Dr. Julia Getzelman reminds her patients, "The womb is the ultimate life-giving and life-sustaining environment. When we think about the effects from a child's environment, the womb is perhaps the most influential."

....

The Immune System During Pregnancy

Your immune system exists to recognize and fight the invasion of an outside organism. That organism could be a pathogen, a toxic substance, or a new organ. For example, people who receive lung transplants stay on immunosuppressant drugs for the rest of their lives so that their body doesn't reject the new lung.

Pregnancy is a bit different. It's what's called a *natural transplant,* meaning that an organism totally separate from the mother—carrying DNA from both mother and father—is *encouraged* to grow in the womb. When you have a developing embryo and then a fetus inside you, your body undergoes a natural immunosuppression. The mother's immune system dials down certain aspects to avoid rejecting the fetus and amps up other aspects to protect both her and the baby from infections. To achieve this balance, Team 2 immunity is activated and Team 1 immunity is suppressed. Team 2, which creates allergic responses, increases locally during pregnancy. This effect is called *Th2 skewing*.[1] If skewing doesn't happen the way it should and a woman retains a normal (or nonpregnant) balance of Th1 immunity, she is more likely to experience problems in pregnancy such as miscarriage, preeclampsia, or preterm birth.

The increased Team 2 activity is not found throughout the mother's body, but it is pronounced right at the interface with the placenta. Certain pregnancy hormones such as progesterone also promote Team 2 immunity. The Th2 skew remains with the baby through gestation and after birth, eventually balancing fully in toddlerhood. Th2 skewing keeps the fetus alive and protects it from the mother's immune system, which might otherwise reject it.

Interestingly, Th2 skewing is strongest in a first pregnancy. Firstborn children are also most likely to develop allergic disease. Babies who are born preterm—and theoretically have less Th2 skewing—are less likely to develop allergic disease, while babies born post-term are more likely to have problems with allergies. This correlation suggests—once again—how interrelated a child's developing immune system is with their mother's.

When I was pregnant with Leo, I had never heard of the Th2 skew. During pregnancy I stopped drinking, stayed away from unpasteurized cheese and fish high in mercury, and made sure not to go into the anaerobic zone during my workouts. But never once did I worry if my daily activities were priming my baby for a more pronounced Th2 skew.

Given the natural Th2 skew and the delicate immune balance of pregnancy, reducing the risk of immune dysfunction *after* birth should start with reducing immune disruption *during gestation.* When babies are born, they have an overly sensitive immune system, which leaves them prone to developing allergic disease. While the immunology of pregnancy hasn't changed in the last fifty years, it's clear that in utero exposures that may affect a baby during their Th2 skew—and the state of the microbiome that the baby inherits from their mother—have changed and made the tendency toward allergic disease worse. These exposures include infections, chemicals, medications, certain allergic triggers, and more.

> In utero exposures and the microbiome that the baby inherits from their mother have changed and made the tendency toward allergic disease worse.

The Risk of Infections

Several studies have shown that microbial infections during pregnancy are important risk factors for miscarriage, preeclampsia, and premature[2] delivery ostensibly because they overstimulate the mother's immune system to the point that it attacks the fetus as well as the infection.

An infection during pregnancy can have repercussions beyond the health and stability of the pregnancy and the birth, too. Even if a pathogen does not infect the baby, the level of the mother's inflammatory response can affect the development of the fetal brain and circulatory system.[3] Down the road, this may increase the risk that the child will develop schizophrenia, autism, and mental disorders. Another study found that intestinal microbial infections in pregnant women can activate immune cells, causing them to cross through the placental barrier and enter into the fetus, forming plaque in the brain. The development of this plaque can lead to a number of diseases, including autism.[4]

The risk to a baby from infections is highest in the first trimester, during the earliest stages of development. Yet it's been my experience that few books explain this clearly to mothers-to-be. Other books may caution against gardening because exposure to dirt can lead to a *Listeria* infection (a bacterial infection that can pass from the mother to the fetus and cause miscarriage, preterm birth, low birth weight, or fetal death) and may warn you to treat a sexually transmitted disease (like gonorrhea or chlamydia, which may cause a child to develop eye infections or become blind). But other baby books skirt around the idea of avoiding infections because the concept infantilizes a mother. Or if they do mention it, they understate the impact of infections on fetal development.

The issue of infections during pregnancy should not be controversial or understated. In fact, avoiding them is an effective and hopefully easy thing to do—for the mother's sake and for that of the child she's carrying. If you're pregnant, don't spend time with people who are sick. Wash your hands often for at least twenty seconds—and always right before you eat—and avoid touching your face. Do not eat raw or uncooked foods that could carry pathogens. Get a flu vaccine if it is flu season, and make sure anyone you live with or spend time in close contact with is also vaccinated against the flu to protect you. Some states even offer vaccines against diphtheria, tetanus, and pertussis during pregnancy as a new strategy to reduce the risk of infection in mothers and babies.

....

The Danger of Chemicals

More and more studies are showing that maternal exposures to certain chemicals—especially those you breathe in—can increase the risk of allergic disease. One study noted that the children of bakers, pastry cooks, and confectionery makers, dental assistants, electrical and electronic assemblers, sewers and embroiderers, and bookbinders and related workers[5]—all jobs that expose pregnant workers to chemicals and dust they can inhale—were more likely to develop allergic disease. Additionally, research showed that a mother's exposure to latex and biocide/fungicide during pregnancy increased the likelihood of wheezing in her children.[6] One possible explanation for this is that exposure to certain airborne chemicals—even at low levels—can cause the body to send "danger" signals that increase Team 2 immune responses in the fetus.

Pre- and postnatal exposure to household cleaning chemicals is also associated with the development of an infant Team 2 immune bias, and house painting has been identified as a risk factor for developing early eczema.[7] Everyone knows how strong wet paint smells. That odor is due to the fact that wet wall paint releases volatile chemicals that an expectant mother can easily breathe in.

When I think about how I oversaw the painting of our entire house while I was pregnant, allowing myself to breathe in fumes that may have led to my son's eczema, I feel terrible. Yet, like me, so many excited parents turn an office into a nursery, then repaint that same room lovingly by hand. Transforming a house for two into a home for three (or more) feels like such an act of familial love, but parents-to-be need to know how dangerous it can be for the fetus. Expectant mothers should engage someone else to do the painting, make them use low-VOC (less than 50 grams per liter) paint, and stay out of the house until the paint dries. During painting, they should ask the painters to open all the windows and ventilate the entire house with fans or air filters as well so the fumes don't stick to bedding or couches.

Chemicals are everywhere, though, not just in paint. Mothers are constantly exposed to chemicals and fragrances in personal care products, drugs, processed foods, perfumes, and bleaches. If there was ever a time to go au naturel and let your pregnancy glow show, it's during those months. Remember that almost everything you put on your skin ends up in your bloodstream, from makeup to sunscreen. None of these products have been tested for fetal effects, and much like food additives, most have been approved under the "generally accepted as safe until we figure out they aren't" classification.

For mothers working certain jobs—like the bakers, dental assistants, and electrical assemblers described above—taking time off while pregnant may be impossible. But perhaps these moms-to-be can wear face coverings during work or change their roles to reduce exposures to inhaled flours or chemicals. Pregnant women may want to avoid cleaning products (make your partner do it!) or switch to more natural products. And finally, go as chemical-free as possible with soaps, shampoos, toothpaste, makeup, and any other personal care products. Anything that smells like flowers or the outdoors but manifestly isn't either needs to be vetted.

....

Avoiding Maternal Allergic Triggers During Pregnancy

I mentioned before that a family history of allergic disease increases the risk of allergic disease in a baby. But the mother's influence—rather than the father's—appears to be the stronger association. In addition, the severity of the allergic disease and the number of flares the mother has during her pregnancy are associated with the development of eczema and asthma in her child. Scientists hypothesize that if a mother's asthma is repeatedly triggered during pregnancy, the baby—who is already Th2 skewed—is exposed to even more immune activity and possibly even the antigens from their mother. As such, avoiding your allergic triggers—like foods, smoke, dog or cat hair, pollen, or perfumes—may help reduce the risk of your baby developing an allergic disease.

Avoiding your allergic triggers—like foods, smoke, dog or cat hair, pollen, or perfumes—may help reduce the risk of your baby developing an allergic disease.

....

Healthy Habits Lead to a Healthy Microbiome

There is some debate about whether the placenta is sterile (meaning it's bacteria-free) or not. Some studies have found oral bacteria in the placenta, while others argue that any bacteria found is due to contamination from the biopsy that's used to gather a sample of the placenta for testing.[8]

If it *is* true that bacteria can be found in the placenta from an internal rather than an external source (like a biopsy), it's still not totally clear how they managed to get there. There are two possible routes, though. The first is through the blood in the umbilical cord. In that situation, bacteria would enter the mother's blood either through the oral cavity or by passing through the intestine and then transfer into the growing baby through the umbilical cord. Though more research is necessary to back this theory up, in certain studies commensal bacterial species have been found in umbilical cord blood, amniotic fluid, and the mucous membrane surrounding the placenta. The other mechanism through which bacteria could pass to a fetus is if bacteria traveled up the mother's vaginal canal—which contains a rich microbiome—and passed into the uterus. Again, however, no study has been definitive. Given that scientists have found both gut and vaginal bacteria in the placenta and the amniotic fluid, both theories may be possible.

What these studies make abundantly clear, however, is that there are in fact bacteria in the pre-birth environment. That's why it's vitally important for mothers to protect their growing baby's microbiome through these three sources: the mouth, the gut, and the vagina. If a mother has healthy habits, she can help ensure she has the healthiest possible biome through which to pass beneficial microbes on to her child.

ORAL HYGIENE

Mouths can be pretty germy, and it's estimated that up to 10 percent of women aged twenty-five to forty-four may have moderate to severe periodontal disease and gums that bleed when pressure is applied. There is a well-established relationship between tooth decay or periodontal disease and poor pregnancy outcomes, and that's why it's essential for mothers-to-be to have good oral hygiene. You might recall from chapter 2 that the mouth bacteria strongly affect the gut bacteria, and the gut bacteria dramatically alter our immune system and responses.

While a meta-analysis showed no clear conclusion that treating periodontal disease during pregnancy could impact preterm birth or low birth weight, many doctors believe that by the time the treatment was given, the damage to the baby had already been done. So if you're thinking of having a child, definitely take care of your teeth and gums. Flossing, tooth brushing, and regular dental checkups are important prior to and throughout pregnancy to protect the baby. A healthy oral biome can only help improve your baby's health. In addition, periodontal disease can lead to heart disease, stroke, diabetes complications, and Alzheimer's, which are all bad news for pregnancy and a mother's long-term health.

DIET

When I was pregnant with Leo, I experienced a lot of nausea, and the only things that settled my stomach were Diet Coke and Sun Chips—both of which I found gross before and after pregnancy. During my long drives on work trips, I ate whatever fast food was available, rather than waiting for healthier food like I might have done pre-pregnancy. I didn't binge on ice cream every night or put on a dangerous amount of weight (in fact, I gained about thirty pounds with each pregnancy), but I definitely felt like it was okay to play fast and loose with the food I ate. My pregnant body had needs, and those included avoiding hunger and nausea.

The truth is, I picked the worst time to let my diet go.

A healthy pregnancy diet is key to supporting a mother's diverse, well-balanced microbiome, which in turn will help the child she's carrying. In fact, a 2021 study from the University of Colorado called Healthy Start measured pregnant women's diets and the allergic disease outcomes in their offspring. Maternal vegetable and yogurt consumption was associated with a reduction in eczema, wheezing, food allergy, and rhinitis in offspring, whereas french fries, 100 percent fruit juice, red meat, rice, grains, and cold cereal had the opposite effect.[9] Therefore, a pregnancy diet should be no different from a non-pregnancy diet, and as I discussed in chapter 5, that diet should consist of:

- *Low sugar, high fiber:* Eliminate sodas, refined carbohydrates, and high-fructose corn syrup from your diet and replace them with foods naturally high in fiber like vegetables (not fiber supplements).
- *Vegetables, fruit, meat:* It cannot be stated enough that most of your diet—up to 90 percent—should consist of vegetables and fruit. They should be frozen or fresh and prepared with healthy fats and without excess salt. If you can, limit processed foods, pesticide-heavy vegetables, and meats, dairy, and fish raised with antibiotics.
- *Fermented foods:* The bacteria that make fermented foods are the same as our commensal gut bacteria, so eating fermented foods is like taking a natural probiotic to repopulate your gut with healthy bacteria. Fermented foods include sauerkraut, homemade kombucha, kimchi, pickles, and yogurt.
- *Low to no preservatives:* Processed and packaged foods that contain a long list of chemicals should be eaten in very limited quantities, if ever, as their effects are unknown and unlikely positive.
- *Supplements:* Several clinical studies have shown that green and black tea polyphenols, turmeric, fish oil, and mung bean are associated with improvement in several inflammatory diseases. Magnesium is anti-inflammatory, and vitamin D suppresses inflammatory mediators, increases bone strength, and more. You can find these nutrients and vitamins in your daily prenatal vitamin, in over-the-counter supplements, or in the foods you eat.

Notice that Diet Coke and Sun Chips are nowhere on this list.

Beyond healthy foods that are gut supportive, pregnancy may be a time to consider a probiotic. As discussed in Chapter 5, probiotics should be used if studied and proven for a specific condition. One of the few that has good data is *L. Rhamnosus* taken from pregnancy through breastfeeding. This bacterium has been shown to cut the risk of eczema in infants by 50 percent or more, and may make sense if there is a family history of allergies.

EXERCISE

Many clinical studies support the fact that cardiovascular exercise for a minimum of twenty minutes three times a week helps improve health, including gut health, more than any other drug or treatment available. Cardiovascular exercise can include running, walking, biking, swimming, barre class, yoga, or whatever you enjoy that also elevates your heart rate. Getting into a rhythm or practice of regular exercise may sound daunting, but it can be the difference between a cabinet full of medicine or not.

Cardiovascular exercise for a minimum of twenty minutes three times a week helps improve health, including gut health, more than any other drug or treatment available.

Diet and exercise support the microbiome because the microbes that have been riding along with us for hundreds of generations, creating the balance that keeps us healthy, evolved in an environment where humans were constantly in the sun, rarely had access to sugar, ate mostly vegetables, and were forced to do physical labor. In order for us to maintain a balance with the microbes that control our immune system, we require high-fiber foods to properly feed them and exercise to stimulate, grow, and nurture them. In fact, a recent study shows that exercise can increase the growth of beneficial bacteria and alter the composition of mucus in the gut, which helps the bacteria that live there.

We often talk about certain diets or behaviors as morally, ethically, or socially superior. I grew up eating mostly Indian food, and my parents made meals that were always vegetarian. As an adult, I wanted to be an easy dinner party guest, so I'd eat meat if that's what the host had cooked. But I never liked meat and certainly never cooked it at home. While I never thought my way of eating was somehow "better" than everyone else's, there are certainly non-meat eaters who feel that anything but a strict vegetarian or vegan diet is entirely harmful. People who follow other diets—like low-carb, keto, or a myriad of other plans—may think their way of eating is the best way. In terms of the microbiome, though, this is a pointless discussion. A clean, healthy diet and a solid exercise plan are simply the things that keep us healthy because they are what our bodies and microbes expect. You would not be surprised if your car engine broke down after being filled with vegetable oil—something it is not designed for. Your body—and the way the immune system works to support or hurt pregnancy—is the same. Give your body the clean, healthy whole food it expects.

MEDICATIONS

Very little about how drugs and treatments affect women and babies during pregnancy has been studied because of the ethics of experimenting on pregnant women. In every clinical trial I have run throughout my career in the medical field, we always excluded pregnant women. The thinking was that it makes the study "safer" to run. However, because every other company does the same thing, pregnant women have very little to go on when considering the use of medicines.

Many pregnant women experience acid reflux, and I was no different. My reflux was terrible with both of my pregnancies, and with Leo, Prilosec was my best friend. Reflux is usually treated with proton pump inhibitors (PPIs), like Prilosec, which are prescribed or over-the-counter. PPIs reduce stomach acid, and in doing so may prevent the proper digestion of proteins, disrupt the lining or barrier of the intestines, and change the composition of your microbiome. A series of studies in the last fifteen years have consistently shown that acid suppression drugs are linked to an increase in food allergy, food hypersensitivity, and asthma.

In order to limit acid reflux and a reliance on PPIs, pregnant women should try eating smaller meals more frequently, restricting their diet to foods easier to digest (toast, bananas, eggs), or increasing the intake of green leafy vegetables (which reduce stomach acid). Breathing and certain yoga poses may also help the body create space for the baby, and sleeping in an elevated position may reduce the possibility that acid will bubble up, causing the burning associated with reflux.

If you develop an infection that requires antibiotics while you are pregnant, use them. The proper dosages of antibiotics have not been well studied specifically for pregnancy, but the likelihood of harm from a true infection (like listeriosis or STDs, which I mentioned earlier in the chapter) outweighs any potential harm from taking the medications that can treat it.

If you develop an infection that requires antibiotics while you are pregnant, use them.

Studies show that using different antibiotics for different infections can help clear the infection faster and reduce the number of side effects specifically for pregnant women, so ask your doctor.[10, 11]

There also has not been extensive research on how aspirin and ibuprofen during pregnancy affect a baby's risk of developing a food allergy. At least one study[12] showed that frequent use of both types of painkillers does seem to reduce the diversity of the gut biome, but there isn't strong evidence to suggest women should avoid them altogether. Acetaminophen (aka Tylenol) has a large body of evidence that shows no harm to fetuses. Of course, none of these studies looked specifically at the amniotic or newborn microbiome or barrier dysfunction, but that should still give you some reassurance. In the event you want to avoid drugs, standard strategies to reduce reliance on painkillers are exercise, warm baths, and massage.

A similar message exists for over-the-counter cold remedies. Despite how ubiquitous they are, their use has not been studied specifically in pregnancy, nor with attention to the effect on future immune disease. Given that cold remedies simply mask symptoms, it may be better to treat common colds with humidifiers, fluids, and rest instead of drugs. One word of caution is that something "natural" can still be a drug. Many websites will recommend this essential oil or that vitamin as a natural way to treat a cold. But anything can be toxic to the body at a certain dose. Vitamins, herbs, or other supplements are still drugs if concentrated and taken in large amounts.

Finally, a word on another category of drugs. It is worth repeating that there is *no known safe* level of alcohol—in pregnancy or not. However, many studies suggest that there may be limited harm if you have a single drink per day, especially if you ingest it slowly and with food. Similarly, studies have shown that a small amount of caffeine—no more than three 4-ounce cups per day—has few harmful effects. And I hope it goes without saying: no hard drugs during pregnancy.

....

Treating Vaginosis

Many hormonal changes occur during pregnancy, and because of that, pregnant women are at an increased risk of developing bacterial vaginosis. It's important to treat vaginosis because mothers who test positive for group B strep (which is more likely with vaginosis) prior to labor will be given cautionary antibiotics to reduce the risk of infecting their baby during birth. Intrapartum antibiotics can wreak *havoc* on a newborn's microbiome.

The vaginal microbiome makes up 9 percent of the total biome in a woman. By comparison, the gut is 30 percent. A healthy vaginal microbiome contains mostly *Lactobacillus* species. These bacteria produce lactic acid, which increases the pH of the vaginal tract; hydrogen peroxide, which reduces inflammatory cytokines; and antibacterials, which prevent infection. The absence of *Lactobacillus* is the biggest cause of bacterial vaginosis. Without our ride-or-die *Lactobacillus*, infectious and toxin-producing bacteria overgrow and the local pH changes, which then allows yeast to grow.

To specifically treat vaginal dysbiosis (or bacterial vaginosis), you have two options. The medically established method is to use an antibiotic such as clindamycin, which will knock out the incorrect bacteria's overgrowth and allow the lactobacilli to reclaim their space. Clindamycin is usually given as a cream that can be inserted into the vaginal tract with a plastic tube. Suppositories—which you can insert with your fingers or with a tube—may also be available.

However, we have discussed at length the problems with overusing antibiotics. You may want to try finding a licensed naturopathic doctor (ND) or functional medicine MD who can help diagnose the problem and give you effective treatments like studied probiotics.[13]

Another "probiotic" method that has been reported to work but is less rigorously studied is applying plain live-culture yogurt to the genital area. It may sound strange, but yogurt is full of lactobacilli, so using it locally is essentially like adding a probiotic of the bacteria you want right at the site of the body part that needs help. If yogurt isn't for you, there are companies that make vaginal probiotic suppositories, which effectively do the same thing. Other studied mechanisms for reducing vaginosis are oral and vaginal treatments of garlic[14] and vitamin C.[15]

Finally, stay away from douches before, during, and after pregnancy. Not only are they unnecessary because the vagina isn't—by its nature—unclean or "not fresh," but douching with store-bought products has been shown to *increase* the risk of vaginosis.

....

Identifying Dysbiosis

Your microbiome, which you will pass on to your baby, can play a big role in the trajectory of their immune development. Unless you have diagnosed issues like IBD or severe eczema, you may have no idea what state your own microbiome is in. Pregnant women have a lot at stake, so it is critical—for their health and their developing baby's—to recognize the signs of dysbiosis and chronic inflammation.

Dysbiosis is characterized by pain, fatigue and insomnia, mental disorders (depression, anxiety), gut complications (constipation, diarrhea, acid reflux), weight gain, and frequent infections.[16] Unfortunately, as of this writing in 2021, there are no accurate tests for dysbiosis, and there is no definition of a "correct" skin or gut biome. As you know, a good or healthy microbiome can look very different from person to person, and among the populations in the world with no allergic and autoimmune disease, people exhibit more variation in microbe species than similarities.

Dysbiosis is characterized by pain, fatigue and insomnia, mental disorders, gut complications, weight gain, and frequent infections.

So how do you know if your microbiome needs improvement or is good today?

The low-tech and gold-standard way to do a self-assessment is to keep a journal of what you eat, environmental factors like pollen levels, and your menstrual cycle. The goal of a journal is to be able to see patterns—for example, "I always feel ill the day after eating tomatoes" or "My skin is incredibly dried out when birch pollen is high." Patterns are hard to see without a well-kept journal because we are all forgetful. But as you take note of certain trends in your health, you may be able to tell if your biome is off or not.

Overall, 15 to 20 percent of people have food intolerances, whereas about 8 to 10 percent of people have food allergies. Food allergies and food intolerances are not the same thing. In a food allergy, your immune system produces antibodies when it encounters an allergic trigger. These antibodies release chemicals like histamine, which trigger symptoms like swelling, hives, or vomiting. A food intolerance is your digestive system's way of telling you that it is having difficulty digesting a certain food, and it causes nausea, vomiting, or diarrhea.

If you suspect an allergy, you can have testing ordered by a physician. In an sIgE blood test, a small sample is taken and tested for the presence of IgE antibodies that are needed for a person to be *sensitized* to a food. You'll get a result for each allergen tested from 0 to 100 kg/IL, with a score closer to 0 meaning no antibodies produced, while a score of 100 means many antibodies. A high test result does not mean you definitely have an allergy, but higher scores in general mean more immune reaction and thus a higher probability of an allergy.

Different levels mean different things for each allergen as well, and it is quite common to see mildly elevated results all around in people who have other conditions such as eczema or asthma. While allergy testing cannot rule *in* an allergy, it can with high certainty rule *out* an allergy. If an sIgE test result is very low, there's almost definitely no allergy. And if you suspect an allergy based on your journal history, then testing can help confirm it.

Remember from chapter 4 that the testing I just described will help you identify anaphylactic allergies only. The stomach allergies and chronic issue allergies that we see in babies are also possible in adults and could be your issue. The only way to identify them is to remove triggers and see if you get better.

If that doesn't work, and you still suspect that something is causing you to feel inflamed, it may be an intolerance. One of the tricky aspects of diagnosing food intolerance is that some people are sensitive not to the food itself but to an additive or preservative in the food or an ingredient used in the preparation of the food. That's not the case with a food allergy, so different brands, washing techniques, or preparations won't make a difference in food allergies if the protein to which you are allergic is still present.

Unfortunately, there are no tests that are clinically useful in identifying the source of food intolerances, though many companies will tell you they can. Like non-IgE allergies, the current best method to diagnose intolerance is an elimination diet. You simply remove suspected foods from your diet completely for about two weeks and see if you feel better. If you do, you add the foods back into your diet one at a time and see what happens.

....

The Role of the Microbiome in Fertility and Successful Pregnancy

A close friend of mine struggled for years to conceive, and over the course of that time she and her husband tried in vitro fertilization (IVF) five times. With the accompanying hormone fluctuations and constant appointments and then crushing disappointment, each round was physically and emotionally exhausting for them. I visited my friend one day, and she showed me the piles and piles of used syringes from drugs she had to inject every single day over more than a year. I've been known to faint around needles, and this was . . . disturbing.

None of it made any sense to me, either. My friend was in her early thirties and healthy. She had a good egg reserve and no conditions that might impede fertility, like fibroids or polycystic ovary syndrome (PCOS). We began chatting about others we knew who had similar, if not quite as bad, experiences, and we found ourselves wondering why stories like hers are becoming increasingly common.

The CDC's 2017 National Survey of Family Growth showed that among surveyed married U.S. women ages fifteen to forty-four years, an estimated 8.8 percent were infertile, defined as failing to become pregnant after one year of trying with the same partner. Over 16 percent of all women fifteen to forty-four years of age had impaired fecundity,[17] meaning difficulty getting pregnant or carrying a child to term. These two categories are a shocking *30 percent increase* from the same findings in 2002. Many people assume this is because the age of women at their first pregnancy has increased, but the age of first pregnancy has nudged up only a year or so in that time.

The truth of the matter is that many of the issues women—and men—face that result in lower rates of pregnancy can also be attributed to changes in our immune systems.

Pregnancy involves building an entire human being from scratch, and that's a taxing process that takes a toll on a woman. As I have mentioned, during a pregnancy your immune system undergoes a number of adaptations to allow you to stay healthy and keep the baby healthy. The immune system also has mechanisms built in to reject pregnancy if the body can't handle it. Women who are too underweight to sustain a pregnancy will stop producing estrogen, lose their menstrual cycle, and stop ovulating.[18] Many athletes who push their bodies to extremes will experience infertility. Interestingly, obesity can also cause infertility by affecting the oocyte (freshly fertilized egg) and causing inflammation in the uterus that keeps it from implanting.[19]

Bacterial vaginosis had long been known to be associated with late-term fetal loss and preterm birth. Now several studies show that vaginosis is also a leading cause of infertility. Up to 40 percent of patients undergoing IVF cycles have abnormal vaginal microbiomes. Studies show that in the presence of strep and other bacteria that fail to produce hydrogen peroxide, IVF success was cut in half. A healthy vaginal microflora at the time of embryo transfer is an important factor in the success of the IVF, and a vaginal microbiome composed highly of lactobacilli is most likely to be successful.[20]

Bacterial vaginosis appears to affect two critical hormones for conception and pregnancy: estrogen and progesterone.

Bacterial vaginosis had long been known to be associated with late-term fetal loss and preterm birth. Now several studies show that vaginosis is also a leading cause of infertility.

An unhealthy microbiome reduces estrogen levels, which negatively affects ovulation rates. It also reduces a woman's progesterone level, which is essential for successful implantation and maintenance of a pregnancy. Progesterone makes the lining of the uterus receptive to implantation.[21] With dysbiosis of the vagina, the uterus becomes progesterone-resistant and inflamed, decreasing the odds of successful implantation.[22]

Polycystic ovary syndrome (PCOS), a common endocrine disease that occurs when cysts form on a woman's ovaries, affects 8 to 13 percent of women of reproductive age. PCOS leads to irregular menstrual cycles, infrequent or skipped ovulation, and increased testosterone levels. About half of women with PCOS are obese or insulin resistant.[23] The cause of this isn't entirely clear, but a number of studies have shown that women with PCOS have decreased diversity of bacteria in their gut and share the types of gut biomes most often found in obese individuals.

The upside of dysbiosis-driven infertility is that it is very solvable in a way that "I'm too old" is not. While I was writing this book, another close friend confided that she, too, had been trying unsuccessfully for months to conceive. We have known each other for twenty years but had never had the kind of relationship in which we freely discussed our reproductive tracts. Yet here we suddenly were, and I told her that I'd just done some research into the fact that her trouble might be caused—or at least not helped—by undiagnosed vaginosis. She heard me out and offered that this supposition might have some merit, since she suffered from frequent urinary tract infections. While this is by no means an example of a controlled clinical study, she tried some of the techniques I've described in this chapter and called the next month to tell me she was pregnant.

....

In Conclusion

During pregnancy, a fetus is bathed in a stew of the immune cells that are involved in allergic disease. This stew is what allows the baby to grow without being rejected by the mother's immune system. And while the jury is still out, there is a fair chance that babies already have a microbiome in utero. In order to reduce the risk that their babies will suffer from an overactive immune system once they're born, women should make choices that regulate their own immune system and maintain a healthy microbiome during pregnancy.

Together, these choices are part of a process that Dr. Getzelman calls "greening the womb." Dr. Getzelman asks, "What if every woman knew that the nine months of fetal life play a vital role in determining her baby's lifelong health? What we eat during pregnancy and put on our skin, whether and how we move our bodies, that having meaningful relationships and a sense of purpose really impact our babies' health, for their lifetime? This isn't meant to guilt trip but to empower women to see this as an opportunity to give their baby the best chance possible for a long and healthy life."

Some of these choices are easier to make than others. Most of us cannot change the nature of our work, but we can avoid chemicals in our personal care routine. We may not be able to limit exposures from food, but we can choose a diet that is 90 percent vegetables and fruit. We can choose which over-the-counter medications to take, reduce our use of unnecessary antibiotics, and use probiotics to maintain a lactobacillus-heavy vaginal microbiome. Hopefully, you'll find these decisions even easier than giving up that last glass of wine with dinner.

I will never know for sure that the choices I made during my pregnancy with Leo—like using Prilosec, drinking Diet Coke, and painting my house—directly increased Leo's propensity for disease. But I certainly would have done things differently had I known the risks. When I was pregnant with Kaden, my reflux started immediately and was at its worst when I worked out, but I didn't rush to the drugstore for Prilosec. Instead, I accepted that I couldn't "still be me." I then compromised and switched from Boot Camp to walking. My reflux cleared immediately. I listened when my body said to stop, and I ended up having a less medicated, less toxic pregnancy.

CHAPTER EIGHT

Biome Care at Birth

Common Misconception:
Newborns need antibiotic drops to prevent blindness.

....

A lot of hospitals will apply erythromycin, an antibiotic, to your baby's eyes within two hours of their birth. The antibiotics usually come in the form of eye drops or an ointment, and they are intended to prevent blindness in babies from STDs like chlamydia and gonorrhea. If you currently have a sexually transmitted disease, your baby should definitely get the antibiotics. However, if you have tested negative for STDs and have no reason to believe that you acquired one between the test and childbirth, you should feel free to refuse the antibiotics.

Like any overprepared type A first-time mom, I had a birth plan written out for Leo's delivery. I'd had an uncomplicated pregnancy, free of anything that would classify me as high risk, so my goal was to avoid these four things: an induction (complete with Pitocin to kick-start or speed up labor), antibiotics (to prevent infection), an epidural (for pain during labor and pushing), and a cesarean section. It seemed like the recovery from a C-section would be much worse than a vaginal delivery, and I'd heard horror stories about Pitocin causing excruciating labor.

After seven years spent in many operating rooms for work, I was also suspicious of any doctor's ability to place the thick epidural needle perfectly into the thin spinal canal. Epidurals can have many nasty long-lasting side effects if the medication leaks internally, including numbness, tingling, weakness, back pain, and more. I knew that while the spinal canal is easy enough to hit if you are very still, I imagined that it would be hard not to wiggle during contractions. (Please know that these fears were somewhat irrational. The rate of side effects is quite low. Doctors are skilled and have had a lot of practice, and they time the injection to a lull in contractions. Pregnancy wasn't my most rational time.)

Leo's birth all went according to plan. Because I decided to take some time off close to my due date, I was working from home when I went into labor in the afternoon. I recall ending an email to a colleague with "I think I'm in labor, so if I don't respond by tomorrow, that's why."

I took a deep breath, called our doula, and started noting the length and time between the contractions. As my contractions got more intense and closer together in the evening, I sent Scott out to get takeout. I sat down to watch my favorite movie, then stood up and paced around the house when I got restless or when a contraction started. I had a good relationship with our doula, so I also diligently texted her every few hours to let her know how I was.

Around midnight I hit the magic 5-1-1 rule (contractions five minutes apart, lasting for one minute, for one hour or longer). I woke Scott up and said confidently, "It's time to go!"

He called our doula, and she agreed to meet us at our hospital.

I don't remember much about the next few hours other than that it hurt, the staff had rhyming names (Vicky, Nikki, and Ricki), and I had to keep my eyes shut so that I could concentrate on labor and pushing the baby out. But five hours later, we had a healthy son, born without medications or interventions.

As is true with most mothers, my birth planning stopped pretty much the moment he was born. I had not thought through the myriad of decisions that hit after labor is over and you're holding a new life in your arms whose care and nurturing is almost entirely—and terrifyingly—up to you. Due to the lack of information out there for brand-new parents, I inadvertently made mistakes that would have helped him establish a healthy skin and gut biome, fortify his barriers, and prevent the development of immune disease.

The goal of your birth plan is to help you communicate (and remember!) your wishes at a very fragile and exhausting moment in your life. The information in this chapter is designed to help expectant parents weigh the benefits and costs of different choices, make a plan for the day their child is born that extends through the hospital stay, and best protect their baby.

....

The Benefits of Vaginal Birth

For most of recorded history, cesarean sections were incredibly risky operations that caused infections, shock, and sudden bleed-outs and were performed only as an absolute last resort. But around 1920, with the advent of anesthesia and an understanding of bacteriology and infections, C-sections became more routine. Then they became positively commonplace. Coming from a recent low in 1997, the percent of cesarean births increased through 2010, and in 2019, they comprised a full 31.7 percent of all births.[1]

That is far too many. Dr. Anjali Martinez, an assistant professor of obstetrics and gynecology at George Washington University, notes: "Cesarean delivery is an important part of modern obstetric care, but the ideal cesarean rate to maximize maternal and neonatal health is likely close to the World Health Organization goal of 15 percent."

Now that we have a greater understanding of the microbiome, the critical role of vaginal birth in its transfer, and an increased incidence of allergic disease, many doctors strongly believe that C-sections should be employed only in cases in which they are absolutely necessary.

Although a baby's microbiome changes over time, doctors understand that the microbiome seeding that happens during vaginal birth is central to the prevention of allergic and autoimmune disease. Science backs this up: compared to babies born vaginally, those born via C-section are more likely to develop immune-related disorders like allergic disease, inflammatory bowel disease, and obesity.[2] A recent study showed that babies born via C-section are missing *Bacteroides* species[3] critical to proper immune development, and interestingly, this problem is most pronounced in people of Asian descent.

Children who were born by cesarean birth also have fecal microbiomes that are distinctly different from those of children who were born vaginally. Their microbiomes are less similar to their mother's gut

> Although a baby's microbiome changes over time, doctors understand that the microbiome seeding that happens during vaginal birth is central to the prevention of allergic and autoimmune disease.

biomes and more similar to their mother's skin biomes. Remember that there isn't technically a "correct" biome, but there is one that your body expects. While skin bugs are great on the skin, the gut needs different bugs for the immune system to develop properly.

There are several steps in the vaginal birth process that may affect seeding of an infant's microbiome. As was discussed in the last chapter, a fetus may already be exposed to the mother's oral microbes because they can be found in the placenta and the amniotic sac. As babies move down through the vaginal canal—usually head down and facing backward—they ingest part of the mother's vaginal biome. Ideally, they also take in some of her fecal biome, because most women will poop during labor, depositing some of it right near the vagina. The fecal microbes come directly from a mother's colon, and as the baby swallows and passes them into their own intestines, it is as direct a transplant as nature allows.

The vaginal canal also stretches and deforms around a baby as they pass through, sort of like a latex glove might do. With its high pH and lactobacillus-based infection defense system, the vaginal lining effectively coats a baby from head to toe. A small study[4] compared the microbiomes of newborns in three groups: those born vaginally, those born via C-section, and those born via C-section who were swabbed with the mother's vaginal fluids two minutes after birth. The swabbing procedure involved placing sterile gauze in the mother's vagina for one hour and then wiping the baby's mouth, face, anus, and body with the saturated pad. One month after birth, the study found that C-section babies who were swabbed had gut, oral, and skin microbiomes that were more similar to those of vaginally born babies than to those of babies born by C-section.

Another issue to consider about C-sections is that almost all women who have them get intravenous antibiotics during the procedure to decrease their risk of postsurgical infection.[5] Unfortunately, we all know that antibiotics are powerful, and there's a chance that they may be transmitted to the fetus through the placenta. Even if they don't pass directly, these potent drugs will remain in the mother's circulatory system and will affect the makeup of the bacteria she transfers through her breast milk. Antibiotics also lower counts of *Bifidobacterium* species, which are known to prevent infection in a newborn.

While there's an argument to be made for doing everything possible to avoid the chance of having a C-section (whether that's by not planning one, by choosing to give birth at home, or by refusing Pitocin, which is associated with a higher rate of C-sections), sometimes C-sections are unavoidable. Not every baby can or should be born vaginally. Whenever I became insistent that "there was no way I was having a C-section" my ob-gyn used to kindly remind me that before the advent of C-sections, 10 percent of women died in childbirth. Sure, I had my perfect birth plan, but C-sections are there for a reason.

If you plan to have a C-section (as opposed to having one that's considered an emergency), you have options that will allow you to seed your child's microbiome as much as possible. The National Health Service in the United Kingdom recognizes and honors parents' desire to protect their babies with the mother's microbes, so British mothers who undergo a planned C-section at thirty-seven weeks or later are allowed to bring a sealed pack of gauze squares with them to the hospital. Women insert the gauze in their vagina for at least one hour, remove it prior to the C-section, and then place it in a plastic ziplock bag. After birth, someone can swab the newborn's mouth, face, skin, and rectum with the gauze, which spreads all the beneficial vaginal tract microbes onto the baby. However, women who have tested positive for group B strep, HIV, hepatitis B, hepatitis C, or herpes, or who are otherwise unwell, are not allowed to perform this seeding procedure for risk of infecting the baby.

Unfortunately, the practice of swabbing is still in the research phase in the United States, so it is not prevalent at all. While doctors may be familiar with it, many won't recommend it unless it becomes a part of a specific protocol within a hospital. However, there's nothing stopping you from swabbing your vagina before birth. All you need is some gauze, someone to help you, and a plastic bag.

For a long time, many people favored cesarean births because it created predictability, doctors thought it eliminated many birth complications, and there didn't seem to be any downsides. Even today, C-sections are more likely in hospitals that are hesitant to perform vaginal births after cesarean (VBAC), where labor is heavily monitored, where there's a great fear of malpractice suits, or if there's a higher insurance reimbursement for C-section. When I was pregnant with Leo, I even remember someone telling me to try to have my baby at the beginning of the attending ob-gyn's shift rather than at the end of it because they'd rush me into a C-section in order to get home sooner rather than later. I'll never know whether this could have happened or if it was just another fear tactic about childbirth, but all I know is that pressing for a C-section when it's not necessary doesn't take into consideration the long-term health of the mother or the baby.

The best way to avoid an unnecessary C-section and yet retain it as a safe option is to find a hospital where midwives handle most of the deliveries. It is proven that having a doctor in the room increases the likelihood of C-section, so working with a midwife affiliated with a hospital will reduce this risk, while ensuring that doctors *are available* in case of emergency.

Midwives and nurses are also more likely to create an environment supportive of vaginal birth. They tend to avoid invasive or excessive monitoring and support the most recent American College of Obstetricians and Gynecologists (ACOG) guidelines[6] to allow labor to continue naturally. In addition, midwives and nurses may employ techniques such as frequent position changes to enhance comfort and promote optimal fetal positioning. Proper hydration and nutrition, along with emotional support, can all help women continue with labor rather than resorting to a C-section.

Finally, if you are able to afford it, hiring a doula will likely increase the chance of a vaginal birth. Like midwives, doulas are trained to coach women through labor, utilize positions that will facilitate birth, and help you think through interventions (like Pitocin) that may raise the likelihood of a C-section. A friend of mine was determined to have a VBAC with her second daughter, but her labor stalled out when she was about four centimeters dilated. When the doctor suggested Pitocin, her doula urged her to take some time to think about it. The ob-gyn didn't see the harm, so he left the room, and the doula instructed her to try nipple stimulation first, a technique that can activate or increase contractions. Sure enough, nipple stimulation kick-started her labor, and she got the VBAC she wanted—with the full support and approval of her doctor.

During labor, many women find it easier to communicate with their doula rather than their parents or partners, whose opinions may push them into hasty decisions. The doula may also spend more time explaining options than a doctor would, allowing a woman to feel more empowered throughout her labor.

....

Avoiding Antibiotics During Labor

Sometime during the third trimester—usually around thirty-six or thirty-seven weeks—women are tested for group B strep (GBS). GBS is a normal intestinal and vaginal microbe and is found in 25 percent of laboring women.[7] Of those women with group B strep who give birth vaginally, only half of their babies will be colonized with the bacterium. Unfortunately, one in 2,000 of those newborns will become very sick, experiencing fever or difficulty breathing.

For that reason, women who test positive for GBS will be given intravenous antibiotics during labor—called intrapartum antibiotics. Women whose water breaks early and who haven't begun heavy labor after twenty-four hours may also be given antibiotics to prevent an infection from forming. One 2021 meta-analysis concluded that intrapartum antibiotics decrease protective *Bacteroidetes* and increase unhelpful *Proteobacteria* in infants. Another 2021 paper found a consistent but not statistically significant trend toward all allergic disease, and a clearly increased risk of eczema, in infants who received intrapartum antibiotics.[8, 9]

What's worse, it's not even clear that antibiotics during labor work for newborns. Studies show that nearly 40 percent of babies born with GBS had intrapartum antibiotics, meaning the antibiotics failed to stop the GBS transfer. Further, as intrapartum antibiotic use has increased, more babies are being born with different infections like *E. coli,* and many are developing later-onset infections like yeast infections or methicillin-resistant *Staphylococcus aureus* (MRSA), a Gram-positive superbug that is notoriously resistant to antibiotic treatment.

These stubborn infections are both known side effects of antibiotics.

None of the above should make a mother feel great about intrapartum antibiotics, but the truth is that most hospitals will insist on them if a mother tests positive for GBS. No one wants to lose a baby, even if the chance is minuscule. That's why a mother's best chance of avoiding antibiotics is preventing a positive test in the first place. Vaginal dysbiosis and bacterial vaginosis are the root causes of GBS and other similar infections. As discussed in chapter 7, a mother can defend against these infections by using lactobacillius probiotics, yogurt, garlic, or vitamin C during pregnancy to prevent a positive GBS test. Furthermore, in the absence of a clear group B strep result or other infection, antibiotics during natural labor should be avoided.

> A mother's best chance of avoiding antibiotics is preventing infection in the first place.

....

The Importance of Skin-to-Skin Contact

My childbirth class and doula had told me in great detail about the importance of immediate skin-to-skin contact between a new mother and her baby immediately after birth, so I was eager to hold Leo the first second I could. The nurses and doctor were all for it, too. Even before Scott helped cut his umbilical cord, Leo and I took a good long while to snuggle, get to know each other, and start nursing.

Vaginal birth is a way to seed a newborn's microbiome, but it is by no means the only way. Microbiome transfer doesn't stop at the moment of birth, and by six months of age, many babies born via C-section have microbiomes similar to those of babies born vaginally.

Early skin-to-skin contact is the next most important step that parents and hospitals can take to ensure a healthy infant microbiome. Skin-to-skin contact allows a mother to swab her baby with her own skin microbiome effectively and easily. As the baby nestles next to their mother's breasts and in her arms, this skin-to-skin contact also helps a baby regulate their temperature and blood sugar. Together, newborns and mothers produce hormones that promote bonding and reduce pain and fear, and research shows that babies cry less if they are held immediately.

Not long ago, the practice was to whisk babies away from their mothers immediately after birth for Apgar testing, baths, vaccinations, and blood tests. Not only were these children deprived of skin biome transfer, they were likely held by multiple people and placed on a number of non-sterile surfaces that inevitably transferred non-commensal bacteria onto their skin. Thankfully, today most hospitals will immediately place babies on their mother's chest after birth and leave them there, naked, for several hours before doing anything else like swaddling them or putting them in the nursery.

Skin-to-skin contact allows a mother to swab her baby with her own skin microbiome effectively and easily.

For babies born by C-section, immediate skin-to-skin contact may not be possible. After a C-section, a mother is usually groggy, disoriented, and exhausted, so it may be difficult—and even unsafe—to hold a baby post-surgery. However, many hospitals try as hard as possible to assist with immediate contact because the mother's warmth stabilizes her baby's body temperature and can reduce the risk of their admission to a neonatal intensive care unit (NICU).[10]

....

Breastfeeding Is Key—At First

I addressed the subject of breastfeeding in chapter 4, but babies are hungry as soon as they are born, so it's worth recapping here. After a baby is placed on their mother's chest for skin-to-skin contact, every new mom should allow her baby to "breastfeed," which really just means allowing the baby to suckle at the breast. For those capable of breastfeeding, the very first day's colostrum provides key nutrients, immunoglobulins, passive antibodies, and signaling peptides that protect the newborn infant from infection. For those who cannot produce colostrum, the act of suckling will also pass helpful bacteria to a baby. Even breastfed babies get 5 percent of their biome from the nipple skin.

Also recall that several studies have shown that supplementation with cow's-milk-based formula in the first week can double the risk of a milk allergy, and both a 2012 meta-analysis and a 2019 study found the same result. After the baby is a month old, the script flips: supplementation with formula actually decreases the risk of a milk allergy.

Pediatrician Dr. Mona Amin has helped hundreds of moms through their early decisions. Here's what she tells moms-to-be: "We know that the early days are important in creating a foundation for breastfeeding, so breastfeeding in the hospital would be helpful. If your delivery doesn't go as planned and you take a pause on breastfeeding initially, pumping will become very useful in maintaining a supply to support your breastfeeding journey. The decision is ultimately yours based on your feeding desires."

With breastfeeding, remember that the first day matters more than the first week, the first week more than the first month. Not all women can breastfeed, and no one should be made to feel like a failure. It is far better to feed or supplement with formula than to allow a baby to become dehydrated—or worse.

....

Avoid Early Bathing

Whether they are delivered vaginally or via C-section, babies come into the world covered in vernix caseosa, a greasy, cheese-like substance that coats their skin during their time in the womb. Hospitals used to bathe babies relatively quickly so that they looked nice and clean for their parents. There's nothing dirty or dangerous in the womb for the baby, so the only reason to bathe them at the hospital is for appearances.

Early, diverse microbial skin colonization is important to strengthen the skin barrier, reduce water loss, and properly develop the infant's immune system. Vernix caseosa is made of water, proteins, barrier lipids, and antimicrobial agents, all of which perform these functions. Slowly, the baby's skin and microbiome take over, but unnecessary early washing disrupts this process, and soaps and chemicals can drastically increase the risk of allergic disease.

Life after floating in the womb requires significant adjustment, especially for the skin, which is a baby's primary barrier against the world. Immediately after birth, the skin experiences water loss, pH changes, and significant growth.

Thankfully, today most hospitals at minimum follow the World Health Organization guidelines not to bathe a baby for at least twenty-four hours. But that wasn't the case when Leo was born in 2014. I watched as the nurses bathed him on his first day, and seeing them washing every speck of white gunk off him instinctively felt wrong to me. Nurses scrubbed each of his tiny limbs, and the whole process seemed unnecessarily rough.

As I think back on it, it wasn't just needless; it was probably harmful.

Based on the research I have done about the immune effects of bathing infants on their day of birth, I believe that the National Health Service in the UK has it right. Its advice to new parents is this: "Following birth, the vernix should be left on the skin to absorb naturally. A comb can be used to gently remove debris such as skin flakes from your baby's hair. It is not good to clear a baby's eyes unless a doctor tells you otherwise. If the eyes are sticky, it is best to gently wipe with a cotton ball dipped in sterile water." The National Health Service goes on to advise that there is no reason to bathe a baby for the first two to four weeks, and if you do, don't use anything other than sterile water.

Following birth, the vernix should be left on the skin to absorb naturally.

How to Deal with Antibiotics and Vaccines Administered on the Day of Birth

A lot of hospitals will apply erythromycin, an antibiotic, to your baby's eyes within two hours of birth in order to prevent blindness from STDs like chlamydia and gonorrhea. The antibiotics usually come in the form of eye drops or an ointment. If you have an STD, your baby should definitely get them. Using antibiotics only when necessary also means *using them when necessary*.

However, if you have tested negative for STDs (a test is typically performed at the first trimester and again during the third trimester) and have no reason to believe that you have acquired one between the test and childbirth, there's no real reason for the antibiotics. While some state laws are different, most hospitals will allow you to refuse the erythromycin, and you should.

I'll note that your pediatrician may disagree with me here to be safe. Dr. Amin countered my conclusion to forgo the antibiotics. "Eye antibiotics for baby are benign and there are no risks to applying them. I usually recommend doing it, since there is no risk. Sure, if mom is absolutely *positive* she does not have an STD, these are probably not necessary. But given that the alternative can be an infection leading to blindness, I err on the side of applying them."

On the day your baby is born, the first dose of the hepatitis B vaccine is usually given as well. (The second dose is given at two months, and the third dose at six months.) This vaccine is made by taking one of the proteins from the surface of the hepatitis B virus, inserting that into yeast, and making more antigen proteins. The antigens are then injected into the blood so that immune cells can create antibodies to fight them.

Hepatitis B is transmitted through blood and is a hundred times more infectious than HIV. An estimated one billion infectious viruses are in one-fifth of a teaspoon of blood of an infected person, so exposure to even a tiny amount, such as on a shared toothbrush, can cause infection. This viral infection is known as the "silent epidemic" because many infected people don't experience symptoms until they are much older. Vaccinating against hepatitis B can prevent inflammation of the liver, cirrhosis, or liver cancer.

I talked in depth about vaccines in chapter 4, but I didn't discuss the hepatitis B vaccine specifically. You should know that there is no evidence that the hepatitis B vaccine negatively impacts the developing gut microbiome or that it is linked to eczema, asthma, or allergic disease. On the other hand, hepatitis B infections have been shown to harm the development of the gut microbiome and dynamically change the ratio of Firmicutes/ Bacteroidetes.[11] Any risk of hepatitis B is too much—especially for a newborn—so it's best to vaccinate your child immediately.

There is no evidence that the hepatitis B vaccine negatively impacts the developing gut microbiome or that it is linked to allergic disease. On the other hand, hepatitis B infections have been shown to harm the development of the gut microbiome.

Since the American Academy of Pediatrics began recommending it in 1961, vitamin K shots have also been given to babies on their first day. All babies are born with very low levels of vitamin K because it doesn't cross the placenta well, and breast milk contains only small amounts of it. Lack of vitamin K, which helps the blood clot, can cause unexpected bleeding and can very rarely lead to neurological damage. These risks mean that all newborns need vitamin K from an external source. Vitamin K poses no known side effects for microbiome development or allergic disease, so there is no reason to hesitate. If the thought of your baby receiving a shot scares you, though, they can typically take an oral dose.

....

In Conclusion

There is no "wrong" kind of birth, but if you are able to have a vaginal birth without antibiotics and with minimal interventions, you should. Important microbiome transfer and seeding happens on your baby's first day, setting them up for a lifetime of better immunity.

Having a plan that communicates your desires to your birthing team can help keep everyone on the same page, but by no means should you feel that your dream scenario is the only way to ensure a healthy child. If you go into early labor or need a C-section, or if your baby must go to the NICU, this is not your last chance to work toward a properly balanced immune system. Many things about labor and delivery are out of your control, and you have to prioritize a safe, healthy delivery first. After the day your baby is born, they have roughly 999 days more to develop an immune system and a microbiome, so there are *many* opportunities to turn things around.

Epilogue

One day when Leo was in kindergarten, Kaden's preschool was closed, and I decided to take the day off to spend some one-on-one time with Kaden. We had the *best* day. We hopped on the subway, hung out in Sister Cities Park—a downtown Philly park with a cool splash forest for kids—grabbed lunch at a café, and wandered home when we finally got tired. Those of you with multiple children know how different they can be when you have alone time with them. But there was more to the day than just how revelatory it felt. Not once did I have to worry if the EpiPen bag was overheating. Not for a single moment did I wonder if the splash-pad water would irritate Kaden's skin. And I didn't have to press the café chef for a list of ingredients or worry about what species of tree my son was climbing in.

The whole day was so . . . easy. Once you've spent years wading through mud, you almost don't know how to handle the freedom of just being. When I got home, I cried. It was one of the rare times that I felt viscerally what Leo had missed out on his whole life.

That's when I decided to pivot my approach to Leo's immune conditions.

Up to that point, I had shared our doctors' focus on making do by mitigating Leo's symptoms. I had mostly come to peace with the EpiPen, creams, and inhalers, and we'd finally sold the changing table that held his medications and found space for them in a drawer. While we were never *comfortable* with his illness, Scott and I had started to accept the idea that a "good" day for Leo was just different from a good day for Kaden. We understood that healthy for Leo meant something different than it did for Kaden, and that our dreams for our sons would have to head down two separate paths.

In my heart, though, I didn't want to have two sets of dreams.

Every doctor we'd seen since Leo first got sick had assured me that there was no cure for immune disease, so I never imagined I could make my son's problems vanish forever. But after all the guilt of feeling like I had done this to him—or at minimum, had let it happen—I sure as hell wasn't going to deal with the guilt of not trying *everything* to make it better.

In 2016, when I had first started to look into a "cure" for Leo's allergies, I quickly discovered that most of the available data about treating immune disease focused on immunotherapy. Immunotherapy is a type of treatment—used for everything from cancer to seasonal allergies—that pushes the immune system toward better self-regulation. When it's used as a therapy against a pollen allergy, for example, an allergist will inject patients with tiny amounts of their trigger (in this case, pollen) every two weeks. When it's exposed to these teensy doses, the immune system learns to ignore them or react less to them. Without an immune overreaction—complete with runny nose and itchy eyes—patients begin to feel as though they no longer suffer from seasonal allergies.

Immunotherapy has been moving into the space of food allergies over the last decade. Different companies and universities have been working on methods to expose patients to their food triggers in an effort to train the immune system to become less reactive to those foods. Patients start by receiving a small amount of the antigen. For example, if they are allergic to tree nuts, they may be given the protein in 1/1,000th of an almond. Slowly, over time, the patient receives a larger and larger amount of almond protein until the immune system stops reacting to, say, three almonds. The patient can be exposed through a patch on the skin (subcutaneous therapy), with drops under the tongue (sublingual therapy), or via ingestion of a food (oral therapy).

Through immunotherapy, a small number of patients are eventually able to get their immune system to forget that it had a file on almonds and thus fully tolerate the nut. They can then freely eat the foods they were formerly allergic to.

Most patients, however, are only able to convince their immune systems to desensitize to a maximum of three almonds. Unfortunately, these patients cannot eat more almonds than that in one sitting because they will experience an allergic reaction. Desensitization can still be incredibly helpful because it means that accidental exposures—like going to a birthday party and taking a bite of a cookie containing almond extract—are unlikely to lead to a hospitalization. For a person who is terrified to attend school, travel, or go to a restaurant, desensitization can be life changing. In fact, most food allergy sufferers will tell you that the persistent fear of a reaction significantly affects their quality of life.

Immunotherapy for a food allergy takes real commitment, though. A patient must take a daily dose (not a biweekly dose, as with seasonal allergies) of whatever the trigger is for *years,* resting for thirty minutes before the dose and two hours after it. You cannot skip doses, either, because doing so risks reactivating your immune system. Toddlers, who change their mind every five minutes and can't sit still, are maybe not the right candidates for an immunotherapy journey, so that's why I'd always been hesitant to seriously consider it for Leo.

When Leo was in kindergarten, though, I realized he was starting to grow up. He wasn't a toddler anymore; he was a little boy who could dress himself, read some sentences, and understand how hard it was to be sick. Maybe, just *maybe*, I thought, immunotherapy might be right for him soon.

Starting 2019, Scott and I began working with the doctors at the Children's Hospital of Philadelphia to create an oral immunotherapy (OIT) plan for all of Leo's allergies. I knew that 10 to 20 percent of kids who start OIT quit because of allergic reactions or because they experience persistent stomach pain during their treatment. Each increased dose of an allergen challenges the immune system, and it may flare badly. Doctors do not encourage patients to begin OIT if they are experiencing regular eczema flares or repeatedly need to use a rescue inhaler because both of those symptoms signal an immune system that is overactive.

Leo has never technically had "severe" issues (though they sure felt severe to me), so when he was six, we decided to try our luck. Unfortunately, a month into OIT, everything went wrong. He experienced one day of stomach pain that turned into every day. Eventually, despite increasing numbers of helper medications, for two days straight Leo screamed in pain and begged to go to the hospital. This was the same boy who had screamed *not* to go to the hospital a few years before, so I knew he was serious. We quit. The doctors suggested we could try again in the future, but I couldn't figure out how that would ever be possible. I didn't want to see my child in agony, and clearly Leo's immune system had nowhere near the peace and harmony needed for the challenge of OIT.

Because I am constitutionally unable to wallow in pity, I went back to the drawing board. I knew there was a growing body of evidence that people's microbiomes change while they do immunotherapy, helping to calm it down, and that this is part of why it works. If all the skin care, diet, and environmental changes I had catalogued for infancy and toddlerhood could encourage and maintain the right microbiome to keep children healthy, could those same interventions perhaps "fix" a microbiome and return someone to healthy?

The more I researched, the clearer it became that "fixing" the microbiome and barrier dysfunction is where science was headed. A number of biotech companies and university labs are working on different methods for exactly that. For some, the goal is to return the immune system to rest so that treatments like immunotherapy can be more successful. Others hope that a repaired barrier will simply cure the immune conditions altogether. Of course, I don't want to wait the ten to twenty years their technologies might take to become available.

The truth is, a *lot* of what we can accomplish with medicine can be achieved with less invasive methods. Exercise is clearly as effective as drugs at changing the hormones and chemicals that cause heart, lung, bone, and even mental disorders. Diet similarly can be as effective as a drug at reversing type 2 diabetes. Physical therapy can have outcomes similar to surgery, and psychotherapy can do better than antidepressants. The best thing about using diet, exercise, and therapy, too, is that they have far fewer side effects.

A lot of what we can accomplish with medicine can be achieved with less invasive methods.

So why *wouldn't* we try healing Leo's microbiome, barriers, and immune system with diet and lifestyle changes that are easily at our disposal?

What I am about to describe may sound like a straight path toward a fix, but I want to be clear that it is anything but. There were many false starts, setbacks, and days of frustration and confusion. Sometimes Leo would get so angry at my fussing, tinkering, and restricting that we would end up in fights.

> **Why *wouldn't* we try healing Leo's microbiome, barriers, and immune system with diet and lifestyle changes that are easily at our disposal?**

No child wants to feel like a test subject, and I didn't want to do anything without his buy-in, so I tried to explain what I wanted to do in terms Leo would understand.

"Remember in *Avengers 3* when the Avengers are trying to stop Thanos's army?" I asked him one day. "Well, there are good bugs in your stomach like the Avengers and bad bugs like Thanos's army. Right now, Thanos is winning, and we have to help the Avengers take your stomach back. I am trying to find things out here that can help the Avengers, and once I do, I think you will feel better."

With that awkward science lesson, Leo was on board.

We began at the surface level, with Leo's skin. I had always noticed that my son's skin was much better in the summer and when we went to the beach. Thinking these good results might somehow be connected to warmth and the sun, I started making sure he spent thirty minutes in the sun every day, and once a week or so gave him a bath with Epsom salts, which sorta replicated the ocean. Soon his skin became less irritated and patchy, though it was still red on his elbows and knees.

We then went through every possible combination of steroids and emollients a few days at a time until we found one type of emollient that worked for his skin. Most brands or categories we tried either did nothing or made things worse, but one specific lotion—lathered on him twice a day every day—made his skin feel sort of soft. Unfortunately, he still complained about being itchy, which meant his body was pumping histamine for some reason.

Next, we started looking for allergic triggers outside of the foods we knew he had problems with. We ran an air filter in his room, and he became less itchy. Then we installed an air conditioner with a filter thinking it would be more effective and keep him from sweating and losing water at night. Unfortunately, the itchiness returned, along with wheezing. Apparently, the dry air triggered his skin and activated his immune response.

I started keeping better notes and noticed a pattern: Leo was at his itchiest in the morning, especially after it rained. I tinkered more in his bedroom, changing furniture and swapping out his mattress. Neither helped. Then I removed his fancy goose feather quilt and substituted cotton blankets, and a lot of the morning itching and stuffiness resolved! Soon we were also able to pull the daily inhaler from his medications.

By this time in my research and tinkering I had become convinced of the power of gut bacteria, so I started searching for probiotics and probiotic foods. We tried one pill at a time, took notes, and looked for changes. After consulting with a naturopathic doctor, who recommended a specific probiotic along with a supplement to remove harmful bacteria and fungus from his microbiome, we saw a dramatic difference. Leo's daily stomachaches resolved, and he felt good enough that we switched from his oral antihistamine to a once-a-day nasal spray.

Two medicines down.

I knew I was getting somewhere, so I bit the bullet and finally decided to adjust his diet until I could finally give him an actual "good" day. As I mentioned in chapter 5, every gut-healing diet is basically the same. They each have their quirks, but overall they agree that you should cook everything at home, eat only chemical-free vegetables, fruits, and animal protein, and stay away from foods with sugar, preservatives, and fillers. Leo and I both hate meat, love carbs, and have horrible sweet tooths. But he was willing to change his diet only if I did, too. Reader, this lifelong vegetarian—whose favorite dish is pasta with veggies— became a carb-free meat eater for the sake of her son.

Leo's results were magical and immediate, and I could not believe I had waited so long to transform his diet. I had always believed our family ate really well, and for the most part, we did. But even the sliced bread and chemicals in the organic packaged foods were too much for him. We pulled everything but produce, meat, and fermented dairy out of his diet to stop the damage, and on the advice of the naturopathic doctor, added a daily supplement that helped repair his gut lining.

With that, the last of his medications fell away. His skin stopped itching completely. His nose cleared. He woke up with clear eyes after a full night's sleep. His belly pain stopped. And even the tantrums plummeted.

Today, the only pill Leo takes is a daily probiotic. We keep all his prescribed medications close by, but he doesn't really need them. We hardly ever have to rub lotion on him, either.

Because there are no dysbiosis tests, I do not know and cannot prove that his microbiome has shifted in a meaningful way toward a healthy one. I also don't know how long we have to keep this up before we can allow some things back in. Part of me doesn't care, though. What matters is that he feels good.

What's also important is that because Leo has now reached this state of health, it's possible OIT could work in the future! Now that we have gotten Leo to a place where his microbiome has improved and his immune system is regulating normally (as evidenced by clear skin and clear nasal passages), we feel far more confident that his body will handle the OIT process someday.

While Leo's immune journey is not over by any means, it feels amazing to see him finally getting better. It *almost* assuages some of my irrational guilt for letting him get sick in the first place.

Because, if I'm honest, that's really what this journey has been about. I've used my son's trials and tribulations to tell a story about one parent in hopes of helping other parents live better, happier, and healthier lives with their children. By promoting a healthy, immune-regulating microbiome in your child and strengthening your child's barriers from the beginning, hopefully you yourself won't ever have to wonder what-if.

Afterword: When Your Allergic Child Goes to School, Parties, or Playdates

I can't go a day without being asked at least ten questions about immune disease. I'm not a doctor, so I can't answer everything—nor do I recommend treatment for someone suffering from an immune disease—but over the years I feel fairly confident that I can address some areas of concern.

Without a doubt, the question I'm asked most is: "What do I do if my child has a food allergy and starts school, goes to camp, or has a birthday party or playdate?"

The first thing I always say is, "Relax, it's going to be okay." Because it is.

I'll start with school. Few things strike terror in the heart of a parent whose child has a food allergy more than their child's first day of school. Parents wonder: Will other children make fun of my child for sitting at a designated food allergy table? Will my child take a bite of another child's

> The question I'm asked most is: "What do I do if my child has a food allergy and starts school, goes to camp, or has a birthday party or playdate?"

lunch, ingesting a food that will send them to the hospital? And will the other parents be upset that they can bring only "school safe" desserts to parties and class meetings?

I grew up in the 1980s and 1990s, and I can't remember a single person in my school who had food allergies. If they did, it wasn't a topic of discussion. Children today, on the other hand, go to nut-free schools and sit at designated allergy tables in the cafeteria. In many schools, if a child eats in the classroom and is allergic to a certain food, no one else in that class can bring that food in their lunch box. I heard a story once of a child in prekindergarten whose classmate was allergic to dairy, tree nuts, eggs, strawberries, and gluten, so no one else in the class could eat those foods during the school day. Parents were left scrambling to figure out what they could pack if they couldn't include bread, crackers, and cheese, which are among a four-year-old's favorite foods!

Today, hundreds and thousands of schools across the country have become nut-free to assuage fears about children being sent to the hospital with dangerous allergic reactions. I think this is an unhelpful change. After all, dairy is one of the two most common food allergies in the United States, yet how many schools have gone milk-free?

Not a single one.

Leo started day care after he was diagnosed with his allergies, so our first discussions with his teachers and the day care directors centered around safe foods and practices. Sure, I worried sometimes that he'd eat something he shouldn't, but mostly I trusted that if I packed him a snack and lunch that wouldn't cause a problem, he'd be fine. He was. Plus, to this day, never—not once—have other children, teachers, or parents given any of us a hard time.

Then when Leo went to preschool, he sat at lunch between his two best friends, both of whom brought peanut butter sand-wiches every single day. My son's situation is certainly not proof positive that nut-free classrooms miss the mark entirely, but multiple studies show that banning an allergy-producing food in a school or creating "nut-free zones" doesn't reduce the rate of allergic incidents—but it does create situations in which children are ostracized for something they can't control.

Most children with allergies do not need to sit at an allergy table, and most parents do not have to panic when they send their allergic child to a school that doesn't have food bans in place. These are the reasons why:

1. *There is little risk for anaphylaxis associated with airborne food contact.* While it's true that peanut dust is a real thing, the amount of a food protein that lands on surfaces, hands, lunch boxes, and other objects is probably not enough to cause a significant allergic reaction like anaphylaxis.[1] Furthermore, the amount of dust that hovers in the air is even lower, meaning that while airborne transmission of peanut protein does happen, the quantities of the protein are not significant enough to warrant caution.

   I always tell people that if they are nervous about their allergic child's exposure to peanuts, they should do what allergists recommend. Put a smear of peanut butter on a table and have your child sit next to it for twenty minutes. Watch for a reaction. Do it again a few days later, but let the child get a little closer. Regaining control and reducing a child's fear of something that can't harm them can be empowering.

2. *Banning peanuts in schools has not led to a decrease in anaphylaxis or EpiPen usage.* In fact, in a 2015 study of Canadian children, anaphylaxis reactions were found to occur

overwhelmingly at home. The rates at school were quite low, and such reactions occurred more often at peanut-free schools (4.9 percent) than in schools that allowed nuts (3 percent).[2] Another study of schools in Massachusetts showed that schools that implemented restrictions on peanuts did not have lower rates of EpiPen usage than did schools that had no such policies.[3]

School is one thing, but what's a parent of a child with allergies to do before camp, birthday parties, or other celebrations, when there probably aren't policies in place? I believe the key is to remember that you can't control others or expect them to feed your child healthy food or *not* feed them foods your child is allergic to. When you leave the house for a gathering, the simplest solution is to pack your own food. This entails a lot of extra work that others will probably never understand or appreciate, but knowing that you have safe food will give you—and probably your hosts—peace of mind. Yes, your child may feel left out when they have to eat the cupcake from home rather than the sparkly blue cupcake made with eggs—but bear in mind that children react mainly to their parents' sadness. Remember that millions of children and adults around the world eat restricted diets for religious reasons. Everyone gives them the space to eat within their rules, and you will have that space as well.

Finally, while many children may be innocent and naive, I have realized they know far more than you think they do. A child who has a nut allergy and attends a school or camp that allows nuts or a playdate where there's peanut butter lying around is most likely *not* going to take a spoonful of it on a dare. Kids don't want to get sick, and they fear getting jabbed with an EpiPen. Parents should also understand that children grow up fast, and before you know it, they'll be teenagers who will be responsible for their own decisions. Kids need to learn how to make decisions early so that they can make better choices the rest of their lives.

Again, relax. If Leo and I have made it this far, you and your child can, too.

Acknowledgments

Most immediate thanks go to the all-star team of Sara, Sarah, and Kirsten, who took this from an unwieldy Google Doc to reality with their incredible instinct and patience.

The idea for the book came from my dear friend Betsy, who gently told me that if I wanted to help educate people, I should sit down and start writing. From there it was massaged and encouraged by my sister Meg and other early readers like Michelle and Katy. Oh, and it was named by Brad Stone.

But, of course, it wouldn't have been possible without Scott . . . who makes all the good things possible.

Lastly, I want to acknowledge the scientists, doctors, and advocates who have poured their hearts into understanding the immune system, its diseases, and how to fix them and prevent them. *They* are the ones who do the real hard work to improve the lives of millions.

Notes

Introduction

1. George du Toit, Graham Roberts, Peter H. Sayer, et al. "Randomized Trial of Peanut Consumption in Infants at Risk for Peanut Allergy." *The New England Journal of Medicine* 372, no. 9 (2015): 803–13. doi: 10.1056/NEJMoa1414850.
2. Ruichi S. Gupta, Lucy A. Bilaver, Jacqueline L. Johnson, et al. "Assessment of Pediatrician Awareness and Implementation of the Addendum Guidelines for the Prevention of Peanut Allergy in the United States." *JAMA Network Open* 3, no. 7 (2020): e2010511. doi: 10.1001/jamanetworkopen.2020.10511.

Chapter One: The Rise of Immune Diseases

1. Max Delbrück Center for Molecular Medicine in the Helmholtz Association. "Genetic Causes of Children's Food Allergies." *ScienceDaily,* October 24, 2017. https://www.sciencedaily.com/releases/2017/10/171024110707.htm.
2. Isabel J. Skypala and Rebecca McKenzie. "Nutritional Issues in Food Allergy." *Clinical Reviews in Allergy & Immunology* 57, no. 2 (2019): 166–78. doi: 10.1007/s12016-018-8688-x.

3. Christopher M. Warren, Jialing Jiang, and Ruichi S. Gupta. "Epidemiology and Burden of Food Allergy." *Current Allergy and Asthma Reports* 20, no. 2 (2020): 6. doi: 10.1007/s11882-020-0898-7.

4. Roxane Labrosse, François Graham, and Jean-Christoph Caubet. "Non-IgE-Mediated Gastrointestinal Food Allergies in Children: An Update." *Nutrients* 12, no. 7 (2020): 2086. doi: 10.3390/nu12072086.

5. George L. Armstrong, Laura A. Conn, and Robert W. Pinner. "Trends in Infectious Disease Mortality in the United States During the 20th Century." *JAMA* 281, no. 1 (1999): 61–66. doi: 10.1001/jama.281.1.61.

6. Abdesslam Boutayeb. "The Burden of Communicable and Non-Communicable Diseases in Developing Countries." *Transactions of the Royal Society of Tropical Medicine and Hygiene* 100, no. 3 (2010): 532–45. In Victor R. Preedy and Ronald R. Watson, eds., *Handbook of Disease Burdens and Quality of Life Measures* (Springer Verlag, 2010): 532–45. doi: 10.1007/978-0-387-78665-0.

7. John W. Steinke, Thomas A. E. Platts-Mills, and Scott P. Commins. "The Alpha-Gal Story: Lessons Learned from Connecting the Dots." *Journal of Allergy and Clinical Immunology* 135, no. 3 (2015): 589–96; quiz 597. doi: 10.1016/j.jaci.2014.12.1947.

8. Megan S. Motosue, M. Fernanda Bellolio, Holly K. Van Houten, et al. "National Trends in Emergency Department Visits and Hospitalizations for Food-Induced Anaphylaxis in US Children." *Pediatric Allergy and Immunology* 29, no. 5 (2018): 538–44. doi: 10.1111/pai.12908.

9. Majid Mobasseri, Masoud Shirmohammadi, Tarlan Amiri, et al. "Prevalence and Incidence of Type 1 Diabetes in the World: A Systematic Review and Meta-Analysis." *Health Promotion Perspectives* 10, no. 2 (2020): 98–115. doi: 10.34172/hpp.2020.18.

10. Yuval Itan, Adam Powell, Mark A. Beaumont, et al. "The Origins of Lactase Persistence in Europe." *PLoS Computational Biology* 5, no. 8 (2009): e1000491. doi: 10.1371/journal.pcbi.1000491.

11. Sally F. Bloomfield, Graham A. W. Rook, Elizabeth A. Scott, et al. "Time to Abandon the Hygiene Hypothesis: New Perspectives on Allergic Disease, the Human Microbiome, Infectious Disease Prevention and the Role of Targeted Hygiene." *Perspectives in Public Health* 136, no. 4 (2016): 213–24. doi: 10.1177/1757913916650225.

12. Helton C. Santiago and Thomas B. Nutman. "Human Helminths and Allergic Disease: The Hygiene Hypothesis and Beyond." *American Journal of Tropical Medicine and Hygiene* 95, no. 4 (2016): 746–53. doi: 10.4269/ajtmh.16-0348.

13. Zeynep Celebi Sozener, et al. "Epithelial Barrier Hypothesis: Effect of External Exposome on Microbiome and Epithelial Barriers in Allergic Disease." *Allergy* (Feb. 2, 2022). doi:10.1111/all.15240.

Chapter Two: Meet Your Real Baby

1. David A. Relman. "Microbiology: Learning About Who We Are." *Nature* 486, no. 7402 (2012): 194–95. doi: 10.1038/486194a.
2. Peter J. Turnbaugh, Ruth E. Ley, Micah Hamady, et al. "The Human Microbiome Project." *Nature* 449 (2007): 804–10. doi: 10.1038/nature06244.
3. Lee Mordechai, Merle Eisenberg, Timothy P. Newfield, et al. "The Justinianic Plague: An Inconsequential Pandemic?" *Proceedings of the National Academy of Sciences of the USA* 116, no. 51 (2019): 25546–554. doi: 10.1073/pnas.1903797116.
4. Jared M. Diamond. *Guns, Germs, and Steel: The Fates of Human Societies* (New York: W. W. Norton, 2005).
5. Rachel Mason Dentinger. "The Parasitological Pursuit: Crossing Species and Disciplinary Boundaries with Calvin W. Schwabe and the *Echinococcus* Tapeworm, 1956–1975." In Abigail Woods, Michael Bresalier, Angela Cassidy, and Rachel Mason Dentinger, eds., *Animals and the Shaping of Modern Medicine: One Health and Its Histories* (London: Palgrave Macmillan, 2017), 161–91. doi: 10.1007/978-3-319-64337-3_5.
6. Elizabeth A. Grice and Julia A. Segre. "The Skin Microbiome." *Nature Reviews: Microbiology* 9, no. 4 (2011): 244–53. doi: 10.1038/nrmicro2537.
7. H. Tagami. "Location-Related Differences in Structure and Function of the Stratum Corneum with Special Emphasis on Those of the Facial Skin." *International Journal of Cosmetic Science* 30, no. 6 (2008): 413–34. doi: 10.1111/j.1468-2494.2008.00459.x.
8. Marissa H. Braff, Antoanella Bardan, Victor Nizet, et al. "Cutaneous Defense Mechanisms by Antimicrobial Peptides." *Journal of Investigative Dermatology* 125, no. 1 (2005): 9–13. doi: 10.1111/j.0022-202X.2004.23587.x.
9. Iva Ferček, Liborija Lugović-Mihić, Arjana Tambić-Andrašević, et al. "Features of the Skin Microbiota in Common Inflammatory Skin Diseases." *Life* (Basel, Switzerland) 11, no. 9 (2021): 962. doi: 10.3390/life11090962.
10. Amy S. Paller, Heidi H. Kong, Patrick Seed, et al. "The Microbiome in Atopic Dermatitis." *Journal of Allergy and Clinical Immunology* 143, no. 1 (2018): 26–35. doi: 10.1016/j.jaci.2018.11.015.
11. Sarah R. Wilson, Lydia Thé, Lyn M. Batia, et al. "The Epithelial Cell-Derived Atopic Dermatitis Cytokine TSLP Activates Neurons to Induce Itch." *Cell* 155, no. 2 (2013): 285–95. doi: 10.1016/j.cell.2013.08.057.

12. Olympia Tsilochristou, George du Toit, Peter H. Sayre, et al. "Association of *Staphylococcus aureus* Colonization with Food Allergy Occurs Independently of Eczema Severity." *Journal of Allergy and Clinical Immunology* 144, no. 2 (2019): 494–503. doi: 10.1016/j.jaci.2019.04.025.

13. Juan-Manuel Leyva-Castillo, Claire Galand, Christy Kam, et al. "Mechanical Skin Injury Promotes Food Anaphylaxis by Driving Intestinal Mast Cell Expansion." *Immunity* 50, no. 5 (2019): 1262–75. e4. doi: 10.1016/j.immuni.2019.03.023.

14. Zhan Gao, Guillermo I. Perez-Perez, Yu Chen, et al. "Quantitation of Major Human Cutaneous Bacterial and Fungal Populations." *Journal of Clinical Microbiology* 48, no. 10 (2010): 3575–81. doi: 10.1128/JCM.00597-10.

15. Gerald Pierard, C. Pierard-Franchimont, Piet De Doncker, et al. "Prolonged Effects of Antidandruff Shampoos—Time to Recurrence of *Malassezia ovalis* Colonization of Skin." *International Journal of Cosmetic Science* 19, no. 3 (1997): 111–17. doi: 10.1046/j.1467-2494.1997.171706.x.

16. Priya Nimish Deo and Revati Deshmukh. "Oral Microbiome: Unveiling the Fundamentals." *Journal of Oral and Maxillofacial Pathology* 23, no. 1 (2019): 122–28. doi: 10.4103/jomfp.JOMFP_304_18.

17. Michael May and Julian A. Abrams. "Emerging Insights into the Esophageal Microbiome." *Current Treatment Options in Gastroenterology* 16, no. 1 (2018): 72–85. doi: 10.1007/s11938-018-0171-5.

18. Inna Sekirov, Shannon L. Russell, L. Caetano M. Antunes, et al. "Gut Microbiota in Health and Disease." *Physiological Reviews* 90, no. 3 (2010): 859–904. doi: 10.1152/physrev.00045.2009.

19. Caroline Bearfield, Elizabeth S. Davenport, V. Sivapathasundaram, et al. "Possible Association Between Amniotic Fluid Micro-Organism Infection and Microflora in the Mouth." *BJOG* 109, no. 4 (2002): 527–33. doi: 10.1111/j.1471-0528.2002.01349.x.

20. Maria G. Dominguez-Bello, Elizabeth K. Costello, Monica Contreras, et al. "Delivery Mode Shapes the Acquisition and Structure of the Initial Microbiota Across Multiple Body Habitats in Newborns." *Proceedings of the National Academy of Sciences of the USA* 107, no. 26 (2010): 11971–75. doi: 10.1073/pnas.1002601107.

21. Roderick I. Mackie, Abdelghani Sghir, and Rex Gaskins. "Developmental Microbial Ecology of the Neonatal Gastrointestinal Tract." *American Journal of Clinical Nutrition* 69, no. 5 (1999): 1035S–45S. doi: 10.1093/ajcn/69.5.1035s.

22. Christina J. Adler, Keith Dobney, Laura S. Weyrich, et al. "Sequencing Ancient Calcified Dental Plaque Shows Changes in Oral Microbiota

with Dietary Shifts of the Neolithic and Industrial Revolutions." *Nature Genetics* 45, no. 4 (2013): 450–55. doi: 10.1038/ng.2536.

23. William H. Bowen, Robert A. Burne, Hui Wu, et al. "Oral Biofilms: Pathogens, Matrix, and Polymicrobial Interactions in Microenvironments." *Trends in Microbiology* 26, no. 3 (2018): 229–42. doi: 10.1016/j.tim.2017.09.008.

24. H. Suzuki, K. Iijima, G. Scobie, et al. "Nitrate and Nitrosative Chemistry Within Barrett's Oesophagus During Acid Reflux." *Gut* 54, no. 11 (2005): 1527–35. doi: 10.1136/gut.2005.066043.

25. Ewa Łoś-Rycharska, Marcin Gołębiewski, Tomasz Grzybowski, et al. "The Microbiome and Its Impact on Food Allergy and Atopic Dermatitis in Children." *Postepy Dermatologii i Alergologii* 37, no. 5 (2020): 641–50. doi: 10.5114/ada.2019.90120.

26. Jeffrey Bland. "Intestinal Microbiome, *Akkermansia muciniphila*, and Medical Nutrition Therapy." *Integrative Medicine* (*Encinitas*) 15, no. 5 (2016): 14–16. PMID: 2798489.

27. Ying Li, Zheng-Li Luo, Yu-Ying Hu, et al. "The Gut Microbiota Regulates Autism-Like Behavior by Mediating Vitamin B6 Homeostasis in EphB6-Deficient Mice." *Microbiome* 8, no. 1 (2020): 120. doi: 10.1186/s40168-020-00884-z.

28. Doyle V. Ward, Shakti Bhattarai, Mayra Rojas-Correa, et al. "The Intestinal and Oral Microbiomes Are Robust Predictors of COVID-19 Severity, the Main Predictor of COVID-19-Related Fatality." *medRxiv* preprint posted January 6, 2021. doi: 10.1101/2021.01.05.20249061.

29. Yun Kit Yeoh, Tao Zuo, Grace Chung-Yan Lui, et al. "Gut Microbiota Composition Reflects Disease Severity and Dysfunctional Immune Responses in Patients with COVID-19." *Gut* 70, no. 4 (2021): 698–706. doi: 10.1136/gutjnl-2020-323020.

30. NIH Human Microbiome Portfolio Analysis Team. "A Review of 10 Years of Human Microbiome Research Activities at the US National Institutes of Health, Fiscal Years 2007–2016." *Microbiome* 7, no. 31 (2019). doi: 10.1186/s40168-019-0620-y.

31. Tommi Vatanen, Aleksandar D. Kostic, Eva d'Hennezel, et al. "Variation in Microbiome LPS Immunogenicity Contributes to Autoimmunity in Humans." *Cell* 165, no. 4 (2016): 842–53. doi: 10.1016/j.cell.2016.04.007.

Chapter Three: Antibiotics Change Everything

1. Andi L. Shane. "Missing Microbes: How the Overuse of Antibiotics Is Fueling Our Modern Plagues." *Emerging Infectious Diseases* 20, no. 11 (2014): 1961. doi: 10.3201/eid2011.141052.

2. Rustam I. Aminov. "A Brief History of the Antibiotic Era: Lessons Learned and Challenges for the Future." *Frontiers in Microbiology* 1 (2010): 134. doi: 10.3389/fmicb.2010.00134.

3. Michael L. Barnett and Jeffrey A. Linder. "Antibiotic Prescribing for Adults with Acute Bronchitis in the United States, 1996–2010." *JAMA* 311, no. 19 (2014): 2020–22. doi: 10.1001/jama.2013.286141.

4. Shane. "Missing Microbes: How the Overuse of Antibiotics Is Fueling Our Modern Plagues."

5. Yun Kyung Lee, Parpi Mehrabian, Silva Boyajian, et al. "The Protective Role of *Bacteroides fragilis* in a Murine Model of Colitis-Associated Colorectal Cancer." *mSphere* 3, no. 6 (2018): e00587-18. doi: 10.1128/mSphere.00587-18.

6. Michael J. Martin, Sapna E. Thottathil, and Thomas B. Newman. "Antibiotics Overuse in Animal Agriculture: A Call to Action for Health Care Providers." *American Journal of Public Health* 105, no. 12 (2015): 2409–10. doi: 10.2105/AJPH.2015.302870.

7. Sabbya Sachi, Jannatul Ferdous, Mahmudul Hasan Sikder, et al. "Antibiotic Residues in Milk: Past, Present, and Future." *Journal of Advanced Veterinary and Animal Research* 6, no. 3 (2019): 315–32. doi: 10.5455/javar.2019.f350.

8. Virginia O. Stockwell and Brion Duffy. "Use of Antibiotics in Plant Agriculture." *Revue scientifique et technique* (International Office of Epizootics) 31, no. 1 (2012): 199–210. doi: 10.20506/rst.31.1.2104.

9. Juan Lubroth. "The New Policy of the Food and Agriculture Organization of the United Nations and Its Reference Centres for the Animal Production and Health Division." *Developments in Biologicals* (Basel) 128 (2007): 73–78. PMID: 18084931.

10. Ying Dong, Christian P. Speer, and Kirsten Glaser. "Beyond Sepsis: *Staphylococcus epidermidis* Is an Underestimated but Significant Contributor to Neonatal Morbidity." *Virulence* 9, no. 1 (2018): 621–33. doi: 10.1080/21505594.2017.1419117.

11. P. Kisembo, F. Mugwanya, P. Atumanya, et al. "Prevalence of Ear Infections in First Year Children of Primary Schools in a Western Ugandan Community." *African Journal of Biomedical Research: AJBR* 21, no. 2 (2018): 117–22. PMID: 31938014.

12. Janet M. Torpy. "Acute Otitis Media." *JAMA* 304, no. 19 (2010): 2194. doi: 10.1001/jama.304.19.2194.

13. National Collaborating Centre for Women's and Children's Health (UK). *Diarrhoea and Vomiting Caused by Gastroenteritis: Diagnosis, Assessment and Management in Children Younger Than 5 Years* (London: RCOG Press, 2009). NICE Clinical Guidelines, No. 84. 7. Antibiotic Therapy. Available from https://www.ncbi.nlm.nih.gov/books/NBK63849/.

14. Lars A. Hanson. "Breastfeeding Provides Passive and Likely Long-Lasting Active Immunity." *Annals of Allergy, Asthma & Immunology* 81, no. 6 (1998): 523–33; quiz 533–34, 537. doi: 10.1016/S1081-1206(10)62704-4.
15. Laura L. Jones, Amal Hassanien, Derek G. Cook, et al. "Parental Smoking and the Risk of Middle Ear Disease in Children: A Systematic Review and Meta-Analysis." *Archives of Pediatrics & Adolescent Medicine* 166, no. 1 (2012): 18–27. doi: 10.1001/archpediatrics.2011.158.
16. Yan Zhang, Min Xu, Jin Zhang, et al. "Risk Factors for Chronic and Recurrent Otitis Media—A Meta-Analysis." *PloS One* 9, no. 1 (2014): e86397. doi: 10.1371/journal.pone.0086397.
17. Stephen I. Pelton, MD. (2021) "Acute Otitis Media in Children: Treatment." UpToDate, https://www.uptodate.com/contents/acute-otitis-media-in-children-treatment; Ellen R. Wald, Kimberly E. Applegate, Clay Bordley, et al., American Academy of Pediatrics. "Clinical Practice Guideline for the Diagnosis and Management of Acute Bacterial Sinusitis in Children Aged 1 to 18 Years." *Pediatrics* 132, no. 1 (2013): e262–80. doi: 10.1542/peds.2013-1071. PDF available at https://www.researchgate.net/publication/241696830_Clinical_Practice_Guideline_for_the_Diagnosis_and_Management_of_Acute_Bacterial_Sinusitis_in_Children_Aged_1_to_18_Years.
18. Barton D. Schmitt. "Fever Phobia: Misconceptions of Parents About Fevers." *American Journal of Diseases of Children* 134, no. 2 (1980): 176–81. doi: 10.1001/archpedi.1980.02130140050015.
19. Martin J. Llewelyn, Jennifer M. Fitzpatrick, Elizabeth Darwin, et al. "The Antibiotic Course Has Had Its Day." *BMJ* 358 (2017): j3418. doi: 10.1136/bmj.j3418.
20. CDC. *Antibiotic Resistance Threats in the United States, 2019* (Atlanta: U.S. Department of Health and Human Services, 2019).
21. Sigvard Mölstad, Sonja Löfmark, Karin Carlin, et al. "Lessons Learnt During 20 Years of the Swedish Strategic Programme Against Antibiotic Resistance." *Bulletin of the World Health Organization* 95, no. 11 (2017): 764–73. doi: 10.2471/BLT.16.184374.

Chapter Four: Baby Care the First Six Months

1. American Academy of Dermatology Association. "How to Bathe Your Newborn." https://www.aad.org/public/everyday-care/skin-care-basics/care/newborn-bathing.
2. NHS, UK. "Washing and Bathing Your Baby." https://www.nhs.uk/conditions/baby/caring-for-a-newborn/washing-and-bathing-your-baby/.

3. Carrie C. Coughlin and Alain Taïeb. "Evolving Concepts of Neonatal Skin." *Pediatric Dermatology* 31, suppl. 1, 5–8. doi: 10.1111/pde.12499.
4. Joanne R. Chalmers, Rachel H. Haines, Lucy E. Bradshaw, et al. "Daily Emollient During Infancy for Prevention of Eczema: The BEEP Randomised Controlled Trial." *Lancet* 395, no. 10228 (2020): P962–72. doi: 10.1016/S0140-6736(19)32984-8.
5. Michael R. Perkin, Kirsty Logan, Tom Marrs, et al. "Association of Frequent Moisturizer Use in Early Infancy with the Development of Food Allergy." *Journal of Allergy and Clinical Immunology* 147, no. 3 (2021): 967–76.e1. doi: 10.1016/j.jaci.2020.10.044.
6. Astrid L. Voskamp, Celia M. Zubrinich, Jodie B. Abramovitch, et al. "Goat's Cheese Anaphylaxis After Cutaneous Sensitization by Moisturizer That Contained Goat's Milk," *Journal of Allergy and Clinical Immunology* 2, no. 5 (2014): 629–30. doi: 10.1016/j.jaip.2014.04.012.
7. Murali K. Matta, Jeffry Florian, Robbert Zusterzeel, et al. "Effect of Sunscreen Application on Plasma Concentration of Sunscreen Active Ingredients: A Randomized Clinical Trial." *JAMA* 323, no. 3 (2020): 256–67. doi: 10.1001/jama.2019.20747.
8. Gerard Pierard, J. E. Arrese, C. Pierard-Francimont, et al. "Prolonged Effects of Antidandruff Shampoos—Time to Recurrence of *Malassezia ovalis* Colonization of Skin." *International Journal of Cosmetic Science* 19, no. 3 (1997): 111–17. doi: 10.1046/j.1467-2494.1997.171706.x.
9. National Eczema Association. "Understanding Eczema in Children." https://nationaleczema.org/eczema/children/.
10. N. Pucci, Elio Massimo Novembre, M. G. Cammarata, et al. "Scoring Atopic Dermatitis in Infants and Young Children: Distinctive Features of the SCORAD Index." *Allergy* 60, no. 1 (2005): 113–16. doi: 10.1111/j.1398-9995.2004.00622.x.
11. Pamela E. Martin, Jana Eckert, Jennifer J. Koplin, et al. "Which Infants with Eczema Are at Risk of Food Allergy? Results from a Population-Based Cohort." *Clinical & Experimental Allergy* 45, no. 1 (2015): 255–64. doi: 10.1111/cea.12406.
12. Donald Y. M. Leung, Augustin Calatroni, Livia S. Zaramela, et al. "The Nonlesional Skin Surface Distinguishes Atopic Dermatitis with Food Allergy as a Unique Endotype." *Science Translational Medicine* 11, no. 480 (2019): eaav2685. doi: 10.1126/scitranslmed.aav2685 2019.
13. Pia S. Pannaraj, Fan Li, Chiara Cerini, et al. "Association Between Breast Milk Bacterial Communities and Establishment and Development of the Infant Gut Microbiome." *JAMA Pediatrics* 171, no. 7 (2017): 647–54. doi: 10.1001/jamapediatrics.2017.0378.
14. Malene S. Cilieborg, Mette Boye, and Per T. Sangild. "Bacterial Colonization and Gut Development in Preterm Neonates." *Early*

Human Development 88, suppl.1 (2012): S41–49. doi: 10.1016/ j.earlhumdev.2011.12.027.

15. Leónides Fernández, Pia S. Pannaraj, Samuli Rautava, et al. "The Microbiota of the Human Mammary Ecosystem." *Frontiers in Cellular and Infection Microbiology* 10 (2020): 586667. doi: 10.3389/ fcimb.2020.586667.

16. Shirin Moossavi, Shadi Sepehri, Bianca Robertson, et al. "Composition and Variation of the Human Milk Microbiota Are Influenced by Maternal and Early-Life Factors." *Cell Host & Microbe* 25, no. 2 (2019): 324–35.e4. doi: 10.1016/j.chom.2019.01.011.

17. Eimear Kelly, Gillian DunnGalvin, Brendan P. Murphy, et al. "Formula Supplementation Remains a Risk for Cow's Milk Allergy in Breast-Fed Infants." *Pediatric Allergy and Immunology* 30, no. 8 (2019): 810–16. doi: 10.1111/pai.13108.

18. Tetsuhiro Sakihara, Kenta Otsuji, Yohei Arakaki, et al. "Randomized Trial of Early Infant Formula Introduction to Prevent Cow's Milk Allergy." *Journal of Allergy and Clinical Immunology* 147, no. 1 (2021): 224–32.e8. doi: 10.1016/j.jaci.2020.08.021.

19. Victoria M. Martin, Yamini V. Virkud, Hannah Seay, et al. "Prospective Assessment of Pediatrician-Diagnosed Food Protein-Induced Allergic Proctocolitis by Gross or Occult Blood." *Journal of Allergy and Clinical Immunology: In Practice* 8, no. 5 (2020): 1692–99. e1. doi: 10.1016/j.jaip.2019.12.029

20. N. J. Elbert, E. R. van Meel, H. T. den Dekker, et al. "Duration and Exclusiveness of Breastfeeding and Risk of Childhood Atopic Diseases." *Allergy* 72, no. 12 (2017): 1936–43. doi: 10.1111 /all.13195.

21. Linda F. Palmer. *Baby Poop: What Your Pediatrician May Not Tell You* (San Diego: Sunny Lane Press, 2015).

22. K. W. Heaton, J. Radvan, H. Cripps, et al. "Defecation Frequency and Timing, and Stool Form in the General Population: A Prospective Study." *Gut* 33, no. 6 (1992): 818–24. doi: 10.1136/gut.33.6.818.

23. Amir A. Azari and Neal P. Barney. "Conjunctivitis: A Systematic Review of Diagnosis and Treatment." *JAMA* 310, no. 16 (2013): 1721–29. doi: 10.1001/jama.2013.280318.

24. Teija Dunder, Terhi Tapiainen, Tytti Pokka, et al. "Infections in Child Day Care Centers and Later Development of Asthma, Allergic Rhinitis, and Atopic Dermatitis: Prospective Follow-Up Survey 12 Years After Controlled Randomized Hygiene Intervention." *Archives of Pediatrics & Adolescent Medicine* 161, no. 10 (2007): 972–77. doi: 10.1001/archpedi.161.10.972.

25. Dorothy S. Cheung and Mitchell H. Grayson. "Role of Viruses in the Development of Atopic Disease in Pediatric Patients." *Current Allergy*

and Asthma Reports 12, no. 6 (2012): 613–20. doi: 10.1007/s11882 -012-0295-y.

Chapter Five: The Importance of a Good Diet

1. Kate E. C. Grimshaw, Joe Maskell, Erin M. Oliver, et al. "Introduction of Complementary Foods and the Relationship to Food Allergy." *Pediatrics* 132, no. 6 (2013): e1529–38. doi: 10.1542/peds.2012-3692.
2. George du Toit, Graham Roberts, Peter H. Sayre, et al. "Randomized Trial of Peanut Consumption in Infants at Risk for Peanut Allergy." *New England Journal of Medicine* 372, no. 9 (2015): 803–13. doi: 10.1056/NEJMoa1414850.
3. Michael R. Perkin, Kirsty Logan, Tom Marrs, et al. "Enquiring About Tolerance (EAT) Study: Feasibility of an Early Allergenic Food Introduction Regimen." *Journal of Allergy and Clinical Immunology* 137, no. 5 (2016): 1477–86.e8. doi: 10.1016/j.jaci.2015.12.1322.
4. David M. Fleischer, Edmond S. Chan, Carina Venter, et al. "A Consensus Approach to the Primary Prevention of Food Allergy Through Nutrition: Guidance from the American Academy of Allergy, Asthma, and Immunology; American College of Allergy, Asthma, and Immunology; and the Canadian Society for Allergy and Clinical Immunology." *Journal of Allergy and Clinical Immunology: In Practice* 9, no. 1 (2021): 22–43.e4. doi: 10.1016/ j.jaip.2020.11.002.
5. Tommi Vatanen, Aleksandar D. Kostic, Eva d'Hennezel, et al. "Variation in Microbiome LPS Immunogenicity Contributes to Autoimmunity in Humans." *Cell* 165, no. 4 (2016): 842–53. doi: 10.1016/j.cell.2016.04.007.
6. Noah Voreades, Anne Kozil, and Tiffany L. Weir. "Diet and the Development of the Human Intestinal Microbiome." *Frontiers in Microbiology* 5 (2014): 494. doi: 10.3389/fmicb.2014.00494.
7. Caroline Roduit, Remo Frei, Ruth Ferstl, et al. "High Levels of Butyrate and Propionate in Early Life Are Associated with Protection Against Atopy." *Allergy* 74, no. 4 (2019): 799–809. doi: 10.1111/ all.13660.
8. Robert H. Lustig, Laura A. Schmidt, and Claire D. Brindis. "The Toxic Truth About Sugar." *Nature* 482, no. 7383 (2012): 27–29. doi: 10.1038/ 482027a.
9. Miriam B. Vos, Jill A. Kaar, Jean A. Welsh, et al. "Added Sugars and Cardiovascular Disease Risk in Children: A Scientific Statement from the American Heart Association." *Circulation* 135, no. 19 (2017): e1017—34. doi: 10.1161/CIR.0000000000000439.

10. Magalie Lenoir, Fuschia Serre, Lauriane Cantin, et al. "Intense Sweetness Surpasses Cocaine Reward." *PloS One* 2, no. 8 (2007): e698. doi: 10.1371/journal.pone.0000698.

11. Dorin Harpaz, Loo Pin Yeo, Francesca Cecchini, et al. "Measuring Artificial Sweeteners Toxicity Using a Bioluminescent Bacterial Panel." *Molecules* 23, no. 10 (2018): 2454. doi: 10.3390/molecules23102454.

12. Bérénice Charrez, Liang Qiao, and Lionel Hebbard. "The Role of Fructose in Metabolism and Cancer." *Hormone Molecular Biology and Clinical Investigation* 22, no. 2 (2015): 79–89. doi: 10.1515/hmbci-2015 -0009.

13. Glenda N. Lindseth, Sonya E. Coolahan, Thomas V. Petros, et al. "Neurobehavioral Effects of Aspartame Consumption." *Research in Nursing & Health* 37, no. 3 (2014): 185–93. doi: 10.1002/nur.21595.

14. Victor Markus, Orr Share, Kerem Teralı, et al. "Anti-Quorum Sensing Activity of Stevia Extract, Stevioside, Rebaudioside A and Their Aglycon Steviol." *Molecules* 25, no. 22 (2020): 5480. doi: 10.3390/ molecules25225480.

15. R. S. Rowe and K. J. Rowe. "Synthetic Food Coloring and Behavior: A Dose Response Effect in a Double-Blind, Placebo-Controlled, Repeated-Measures Study." *Journal of Pediatrics* 125, no. 5, Pt 1 (1994): 691–98. doi: 10.1016/s0022-3476(94)70059-1.

16. Environmental Working Group. https://www.ewg.org/foodnews/.

17. Environmental Working Group. https://www.ewg.org/foodnews /clean-fifteen.php.

18. Associated Press. "Bayer to Pay Up to $10.9 Billion to Settle Roundup Weedkiller Case." *Philadephia Inquirer,* June 24, 2020. https://www .inquirer.com/news/nation-world/bayer-settlement-monsanto -roundup-weedkiller-cancer-causing-20200624.html.

19. Anthony Samsel and Stephanie Seneff. "Glyphosate, Pathways to Modern Diseases II: Celiac Sprue and Gluten Intolerance." *Interdisciplinary Toxicology* 6, no. 4 (2013): 159–84. doi: 10.2478/ intox-2013-0026.

20. Alessio Fasano and Carlo Catassi. "Celiac Disease." World Gastroenterology Organisation. https://www.worldgastroenterology .org/publications/e-wgn/e-wgn-expert-point-of-view-articles-collection /the-global-village-of-celiac-disease-and-its-evolution-over-time.

21. Adrian Tett, Kun D. Huang, Francesco Asnicar, et al. "The *Prevotella copri* Complex Comprises Four Distinct Clades Underrepresented in Westernized Populations." *Cell Host & Microbe* 26, no. 5 (2019): 666–79.e7. doi: 10.1016/j.chom.2019.08.018.

22. The Microsetta Initiative. http://americangut.org/.

23. Voreades, Kozil, and Weir. "Diet and the Development of the Human Intestinal Microbiome."

24. Maria Elisabetta Baldassarre, Valentina Palladino, Anna Amoruso, et al. "Rationale of Probiotic Supplementation During Pregnancy and Neonatal Period." *Nutrients* 10, no. 11 (2018): 1693. doi: 10.3390/nu10111693.
25. Kristin Wickens, Peter N. Black, Thorsten V. Stanley, et al. "A Differential Effect of 2 Probiotics in the Prevention of Eczema and Atopy: A Double-Blind, Randomized, Placebo-Controlled Trial." *Journal of Allergy and Clinical Immunology* 122, no. 4 (2008): 788–94. doi: 10.1016/j.jaci.2008.07.011.

Chapter Six: The Impact of the Environment

1. Pajau Vangay, Abigail J. Johnson, Tonya L. Ward, et al. "US Immigration Westernizes the Human Gut Microbiome." *Cell* 175, no. 4 (2018): 962–72.e10. doi: 10.1016/j.cell.2018.10.029.
2. Elina Jerschow, Aileen P. McGinn, Gabriele de Vos, et al. "Dichlorophenol-Containing Pesticides and Allergies: Results from the US National Health and Nutrition Examination Survey 2005–2006." *Annals of Allergy, Asthma & Immunology* 109, no. 6 (2012): 420–25. doi: 10.1016/j.anai.2012.09.005.
3. EWG Tap Water Database. https://www.ewg.org/tapwater/.
4. Batın Ilgıt Sezgin, Sirin Güner Onur, Ali Mentes, et al. "Two-Fold Excess of Fluoride in the Drinking Water Has No Obvious Health Effects Other Than Dental Fluorosis." *Journal of Trace Elements in Medicine and Biology* 50 (2018): 216–22. doi: 10.1016/j.jtemb.2018.07.004.
5. Winifried E. H. Blum, Sophie Zechmeister-Boltenstern, and Katharina M. Keiblinger. "Does Soil Contribute to the Human Gut Microbiome?" *Microorganisms* 7, no. 9 (2019): 287. doi: 10.3390/microorganisms7090287.
6. Winifried E. H. Blum, et al. "Does Soil Contribute to the Human Gut Microbiome?"
7. Lucette Flandroy, Theofilos Poutahidis, Gabriele Berg, et al. "The Impact of Human Activities and Lifestyles on the Interlinked Microbiota and Health of Humans and of Ecosystems." *Science of the Total Environment* 627 (2018): 1018–38. doi: 10.1016/j.scitotenv.2018.01.288.
8. Michelle M. Stein, Cara L. Hrusch, Justyna Gozdz, et al. "Innate Immunity and Asthma Risk in Amish and Hutterite Farm Children." *New England Journal of Medicine* 375, no. 5 (2016): 411–21. doi: 10.1056/NEJMoa1508749.
9. Rie Sakai-Bizmark, Scott M. I. Friedlander, Karin Oshima, et al. "Urban/Rural Residence Effect on Emergency Department Visits

Arising from Food-Induced Anaphylaxis." *Allergology International* 68, no. 3 (2019): 316–20. doi: 10.1016/j.alit.2018.12.007.

10. Brian D. Muegge, Justin Kuczynski, Dan Knights, et al. "Diet Drives Convergence in Gut Microbiome Functions Across Mammalian Phylogeny and Within Humans." *Science* 332, no. 6032 (2011): 970–74. doi: 10.1126/science.1198719.

11. M. E. R. O'Brien, H. Anderson, E. Kaukel, et al. "SRL172 (Killed *Mycobacterium vaccae*) in Addition to Standard Chemotherapy Improves Quality of Life Without Affecting Survival, in Patients with Advanced Non-Small-Cell Lung Cancer: Phase III Results." *Annals of Oncology* 15, no. 6 (2004): 906–14. doi: 10.1093/annonc/mdh220.

12. T. Konya, B. Koster, H. Maughan, et al. "Associations Between Bacterial Communities of House Dust and Infant Gut." *Environmental Research* 131 (2014): 25–30. doi: 10.1016/j.envres.2014.02.005.

13. Lidia Casas, Anne M. Karvonen, Pirkka V. Kirjavainen, et al. "Early Life Home Microbiome and Hyperactivity/Inattention in School-Age Children." *Scientific Reports* 9 (2019): 17355. doi: 10.1038/s41598-019-53527-1.

14. Hein M. Tun, Theodore Konya, Tim K. Takaro, et al. "Exposure to Household Furry Pets Influences the Gut Microbiota of Infant at 3-4 Months Following Various Birth Scenarios." *Microbiome* 5, no. 1 (2017): 40. doi: 10.1186/s40168-017-0254-x.

15. Martin Frederik Laursen, Gitte Zachariassen, Martin Iain Bahl, et al. "Having Older Siblings Is Associated with Gut Microbiota Development During Early Childhood." *BMC Microbiology* 15 (2015): 154. doi: 10.1186/s12866-015-0477-6.

16. Mu Xian, Paulina Wawrzyniak, Beate Rückert, et al. "Anionic Surfactants and Commercial Detergents Decrease Tight Junction Barrier Integrity in Human Keratinocytes." *Journal of Allergy and Clinical Immunology* 138, no. 3 (2016): 890–93.e9. doi: 10.1016/j.jaci.2016.07.003; Ming Wang, Ge Tan, Andrzej Eljaszewicz, et al. "Laundry Detergents and Detergent Residue After Rinsing Directly Disrupt Tight Junction Barrier Integrity in Human Bronchial Epithelial Cells." *Journal of Allergy and Clinical Immunology* 143, no. 5 (2019): 1892–1903. doi: 10.1016/j.jaci.2018.11.016.

17. B. Brett Finlay, Katherine R. Amato, Meghan Azad, et al. "The Hygiene Hypothesis, the COVID Pandemic, and Consequences for the Human Microbiome." *Proceedings of the National Academy of Sciences of the USA* 118, no. 6 (2021): e2010217118. doi: 10.1073/pnas.2010217118.

18. Eric B. Brandt, Jocelyn M. Biagini Myers, Patrick H. Ryan, et al. "Air Pollution and Allergic Diseases." *Current Opinion in Pediatrics* 27, no. 6 (2015): 724–35. doi: 10.1097/MOP.0000000000000286.

19. Teresa To, Jingqin Zhu, Dave Stieb, et al. "Early Life Exposure to Air Pollution and Incidence of Childhood Asthma, Allergic Rhinitis and Eczema." *European Respiratory Journal* 55, no. 2 (2020): 1900913. doi: 10.1183/13993003.00913-2019.
20. Julie Carré, Nicolas Gatimel, Jessika Moreau, et al. "Does Air Pollution Play a Role in Infertility?: A Systematic Review." *Environmental Health* 16, no. 1 (2017): 82. doi: 10.1186/s12940-017-0291-8.
21. Shau-Ku Huang, Qingling Zhang, Zhiming Qiu, et al. "Mechanistic Impact of Outdoor Air Pollution on Asthma and Allergic Diseases." *Journal of Thoracic Disease* 7, no. 1 (2015): 23–33. doi: 10.3978/j.issn.2072-1439.2014.12.13.
22. Adrianna Gałuszka, Małgorzata Stec, Kazimierz Węglarczyk, et al. "Transition Metal Containing Particulate Matter Promotes Th1 and Th17 Inflammatory Response by Monocyte Activation in Organic and Inorganic Compounds Dependent Manner." *International Journal of Environmental Research and Public Health* 17, no. 4 (2020): 1227. doi: 10.3390/ijerph17041227.
23. Kyung-Duk Min, Seon-Ju Yi, Hwan-Cheol Kim, et al. "Association Between Exposure to Traffic-Related Air Pollution and Pediatric Allergic Diseases Based on Modeled Air Pollution Concentrations and Traffic Measures in Seoul, Korea: A Comparative Analysis." *Environmental Health* 19, no. 1 (2020): 6. doi: 10.1186/s12940-020-0563-6.
24. Brian Sawers, *Minnesota Law Review.* "Regulating Pollen." February 14, 2014. https://minnesotalawreview.org/supplement/regulating-pollen/.
25. University of East Anglia. "It's Official—Spending Time Outside Is Good for You." ScienceDaily, July 6, 2018. www.sciencedaily.com/releases/2018/07/180706102842.htm.

Chapter Seven: Nurturing Your Baby's Biome During Pregnancy

1. J. P. McFadden, Jacob P. Thyssen, D. A. Basketter, et al. "T Helper Cell 2 Immune Skewing in Pregnancy/Early Life: Chemical Exposure and the Development of Atopic Disease and Allergy." *British Journal of Dermatology* 172, no. 3 (2015): 584–91. doi: 10.1111/bjd.13497.
2. Ronald F. Lamont. "Advances in the Prevention of Infection-Related Preterm Birth." *Frontiers in Immunology* 6 (2015): 566. doi: 10.3389/fimmu.2015.00566.
3. Mohammed Amir, Julia A. Brown, Stephanie L. Rager, et al. "Maternal Microbiome and Infections in Pregnancy." *Microorganisms* 8, no. 12 (2020): 1996. doi: 10.3390/microorganisms8121996.

4. Sangdoo Kim, Hyunju Kim, Yeong Shin Yim, et al. "Maternal Gut Bacteria Promote Neurodevelopmental Abnormalities in Mouse Offspring." *Nature* 549 (2017): 528–32. doi: 10.1038/nature23910.

5. L. L. Magnusson, H. Wennborg, J. P. Bonde, et al. "Wheezing, Asthma, Hay Fever, and Atopic Eczema in Relation to Maternal Occupations in Pregnancy." *Occupational & Environmental Medicine* 63, no. 9 (2006): 640–66. doi: 10.1136/oem.2005.024422.

6. N. Tagiyeva, G. Devereux, S. Semple, et al. "Parental Occupation Is a Risk Factor for Childhood Wheeze and Asthma." *European Respiratory Journal* 35 (2010): 987–93. doi: 10.1183/09031936.00050009.

7. Amy M. Padula, Catherine Monk, Patricia A. Brennan, et al. "A Review of Maternal Prenatal Exposures to Environmental Chemicals and Psychosocial Stressors—Implications for Research on Perinatal Outcomes in the ECHO Program." *Journal of Perinatology* 40, no. 1 (2020): 10–24. doi: 10.1038/s41372-019-0510-y.

8. Marcus C. de Goffau, Susanne Lager, Ulla Sovio, et al. "Human Placenta Has No Microbiome but Can Contain Potential Pathogens." *Nature* 572 (2019): 329–34. doi: 10.1038/s41586-019-1451-5.

9. Carina Venter, Michaela P. Palumbo, Deborah H. Glueck, et al. "The Maternal Diet Index in Pregnancy Is Associated with Offspring Allergic Diseases: The Healthy Start Study." *Allergy* 77 no. 1 (2022): 162–172. doi:10.1111/all.14949.

10. Dorothy L. Moore, Upton D. Allen, and Timothy Mailman. "Invasive Group A Streptococcal Disease: Management and Chemoprophylaxis." *Paediatrics & Child Health* 24, no. 2 (2019): 128. doi: 10.1093/pch/pxz039.

11. Catherine Cluver, Natalia Novikova, David Oa Eriksson, et al. "Interventions for Treating Genital *Chlamydia trachomatis* Infection in Pregnancy." *Cochrane Database of Systemic Reviews* 9, no. 9 (2017): CD010485. doi: 10.1002/14651858.CD010485.pub2.

12. M. A. M. Rogers and D. M. Aronoff. "The Influence of Non-Steroidal Anti-Inflammatory Drugs on the Gut Microbiome." *Clinical Microbiology and Infection* 22, no. 2 (2016): 178.e1–e9. doi: 10.1016/j.cmi.2015.10.003.

13. Maria Elisabetta Baldassarre, Valentina Palladino, Anna Amoruso, et al. "Rationale of Probiotic Supplementation During Pregnancy and Neonatal Period." *Nutrients* 10, no. 11 (2018): 1693. doi: 10.3390/nu10111693.

14. Farnaz Mohammadzadeh, Mahrokh Dolatian, Masoome Jorjani, et al. "Comparing the Therapeutic Effects of Garlic Tablet and Oral Metronidazole on Bacterial Vaginosis: A Randomized Controlled Clinical Trial." *Iran Red Crescent Medical Journal* 16, no. 7 (2014): e19118. doi: 10.5812/ircmj.19118.

15. Eiko E. Petersen, Margherita Genet, Maurizio Caserini, et al. "Efficacy of Vitamin C Vaginal Tablets in the Treatment of Bacterial Vaginosis: A Randomised, Double Blind, Placebo Controlled Clinical Trial." *Arzneimittelforschung* 61, no. 4 (2011): 260–65. doi: 10.1055/s-0031-1296197.

16. Roma Pahwa, Amandeep Goyal, Pankaj Bansal, et al. *Chronic Inflammation.* In StatPearls [Internet] (Treasure Island, FL: StatPearls Publishing, 2021).

17. CDC Center for Health Statistics. "Infertility." https://www.cdc.gov /nchs/fastats/infertility.htm.

18. M. C. Kimmel, E. H. Ferguson, S. Zerwas, et al. "Obstetric and Gynecologic Problems Associated with Eating Disorders." *International Journal of Eating Disorders* 49, no. 3 (2016): 260–75. doi: 10.1002/eat.22483.

19. Darcy E. Broughton and Kelle H. Moley. "Obesity and Female Infertility: Potential Mediators of Obesity's Impact." *Fertility and Sterility* 107, no. 4 (2017): 840–47. doi: 10.1016/j.fertnstert.2017.01.017.

20. Richard W. Hyman, Christopher N. Herndon, Hui Jiang, et al. "The Dynamics of the Vaginal Microbiome During Infertility Therapy with In Vitro Fertilization-Embryo Transfer." *Journal of Assisted Reproduction and Genetics* 29, no. 2 (2012): 105–15. doi: 10.1007/ s10815-011-9694-6.

21. Linda C. Giudice, Tracey L. Telles, Shalini Lobo, et al. "The Molecular Basis for Implantation Failure in Endometriosis: On the Road to Discovery." *Annals of the New York Academy of Sciences* 955 (2002): 252–64; discussion 293–95, 396–406. doi: 10.1111/j.1749-6632.2002. tb02786.x.

22. Ido Sirota, Shvetha M. Zarek, and James H. Segars. "Potential Influence of the Microbiome on Infertility and Assisted Reproductive Technology." *Seminars in Reproductive Medicine* 32, no. 1 (2014): 35–42. doi: 10.1055/s-0033-1361821.

23. Xiaoxuan Zhao, Yuepeng Jiang, Hongyan Xi, et al. "Exploration of the Relationship Between Gut Microbiota and Polycystic Ovary Syndrome (PCOS): A Review." *Geburtshilfe und Frauenheilkunde* 80, no. 2 (2020): 161–71. doi: 10.1055/a-1081-2036.

Chapter Eight: Biome Care at Birth

1. Michelle J. K. Osterman, B. E. Hamilton, J. A. Martin, A. K. Driscoll, and C. P. Valenzuela. "Births: Final data for 2020." *National Vital Statistics Reports* 70, no. 17. Hyattsville, MD: National Center for Health Statistics, 2022. doi: https://dx.doi.org/10.15620/cdc:112078.

2. Mairead Black, Siladitya Bhattacharya, Sam Philip, et al. "Planned Repeat Cesarean Section at Term and Adverse Childhood Health Outcomes: A Record-Linkage Study." *PLoS Medicine* 13, no. 2 (2016): e1001973. doi: 10.1371/journal.pmed.1001973.
3. Gyungcheon Kim, Jaewoong Bae, Mi Jin Kim, et al. "Delayed Establishment of Gut Microbiota in Infants Delivered by Cesarean Section." *Frontiers in Microbiology* 11 (2020): 2099. doi: 10.3389/fmicb.2020.02099.
4. Maria G. Dominguez-Bello, Kassandra M. De Jesus-Laboy, Nan Shen, et al. "Partial Restoration of the Microbiota of Cesarean-Born Infants via Vaginal Microbial Transfer." *Nature Medicine* 22, no. 3 (2016): 250–53. doi: 10.1038/nm.4039.
5. Fiona M. Smaill and Rosalie M. Grivell. "Antibiotic Prophylaxis Versus No Prophylaxis for Preventing Infection After Cesarean Section." *Cochrane Database of Systematic Reviews* 10 (October 28, 2014): CD007482. doi: 10.1002/14651858.CD007482.pub3.
6. American College of Obstetricians and Gynecologists, et al. "Safe Prevention of the Primary Cesarean Delivery." *American Journal of Obstetrics and Gynecology* 210, no. 3 (2014): 179–93. doi: 10.1016/j.ajog.2014.01.026.
7. Centers for Disease Control and Prevention. "Group B Strep (GBS)." https://www.cdc.gov/groupbstrep/.
8. S. Prescott, et al. "Impact of Intrapartum Antibiotic Prophylaxis on Offspring Microbiota." *Frontiers in Pediatrics*, vol. 9 754013 (Dec. 10, 2021). doi:10.3389/fped.2021.754013
9. Miren B. Dhudasia, et al. "Intrapartum Group B Streptococcal Prophylaxis and Childhood Allergic Disorders." *Pediatrics*, vol. 147, 5 (2021): e2020012187. doi:10.1542/peds.2020-012187
10. Selena Posthuma, Fleurisca J. Korteweg, J. Marinus van der Ploeg, et al. "Risks and Benefits of the Skin-to-Skin Cesarean Section—A Retrospective Cohort Study." *Journal of Maternal-Fetal & Neonatal Medicine* 30, no. 2 (2017): 159–63. doi: 10.3109/14767058.2016.1163683.
11. Quingfeng Zhu, Panpan Xia, Xin Zhou, et al. "Hepatitis B Virus Alters Gut Microbiota Composition in Mice." *Frontiers in Cellular and Infection Microbiology* 9 (2019): 377. doi: 10.3389/fcimb.2019.00377.

Afterword

1. Steven J. Simonte, Songhui Ma, Shideh Mofidi, et al. "Relevance of Casual Contact with Peanut Butter in Children with Peanut Allergy." *Journal of Allergy and Clinical Immunology* 112, no. 1 (2003): 180–82. doi: 10.1067/mai.2003.1486.

2. Sabrine Cherkaoui, Moshe Ben-Shoshan, Reza Alizadehfar, et al. "Accidental Exposures to Peanut in a Large Cohort of Canadian Children with Peanut Allergy." *Clinical and Translational Allergy* 5 (2015): 16. doi: 10.1186/s13601-015-0055-x.

3. Lisa M. Bartnikas, Michelle F. Huffaker, William J. Sheehan, et al. "Impact of School Peanut-Free Policies on Epinephrine Administration." *Journal of Allergy and Clinical Immunology* 140, no. 2 (2017): 465–73. doi: 10.1016/j.jaci.2017.01.040.

Index